JN298444

薬学生のための
実践英語

Communicate Like a Pro:
Practical English for Student Pharmacists

Eric M. Skier・上鶴重美 著

CD付

東京化学同人

まえがき

　本書は薬学部の学生，特に海外研修に参加したり，英語での学会発表に臨んだり，就職活動を始める学生に向けて執筆しました．本書のねらいは，読者の皆さんが英語で"プロらしくコミュニケーション"をとれるようになることです．プロらしい英語コミュニケーションとは，常識をわきまえ，知的で丁寧な表現を使った話し方であり，書き方を意味します．私は長年，日本で英語を教えていますが，日本人は英語を使ったコミュニケーションがあまり上手ではないと思うことがときどきあります．たとえば，不適切な表現を使っていたり，いきなり相手をファーストネームで呼んだり，言うべきときに"thank you"を言わなかったりしています．また日本人は，英語で書く能力（writing skills）や英語を聴く能力（listening skills）が乏しく，英語でのプレゼンテーション能力に至ってはほとんど備わっていません．英語を適切にかつ丁寧に使う能力は，就職活動にも社会人になってからも不可欠です．英語能力をもつ社員を求める企業はますます増えています．

　本書では英語での自己紹介の仕方（口頭や書面）や就職活動における面接者との英語でのやりとりを取上げました．また薬学に携わる人が英語を活用する機会も増えてきましたので，英語でのプレゼンテーション方法のコツなども紹介します．随所の"Eric's Tips"では，日本と英語圏の文化・言語・マナー・服装などの相違について解説します．

　学生のときに教室の中だけで本書を使うのではなく，社会人になってからもいろいろな場面でお役立ていただければ幸いです．

2013年5月

執筆者を代表して
Eric M. Skier

執筆者紹介

Eric M. Skier

1969年米国ロサンゼルス生まれ．2002年コロンビア大学ティーチャーズカレッジ修士課程修了．1994年より日本の大学で英語教育に従事．東京薬科大学薬学部 専任講師を経て，2011年より准教授（英語教育）．日本やカリフォルニア大学をはじめ米国の薬剤師および薬学教育にかかわる人達との交流とともに，日本の薬学生を米国や横田基地の医療施設などに引率した経験をもとに本書を執筆した．専門は英語教授法．剣道5段．

おもな著書："薬学英語入門（プライマリー薬学シリーズ1）"，"薬学生・薬剤師のための英会話ハンドブック"，"看護師のための英会話ハンドブック"（いずれも共著，東京化学同人）

上鶴重美（Shigemi Kamitsuru, RN, Ph.D.）

長野県生まれ．千葉大学教育学部看護教員養成課程卒業．公立病院勤務を経て1989年米国に留学．1991年ケースウェスタンリザーブ大学修士課程修了．米国でも看護師免許を取得し大学病院に勤務．1996年ボストンカレッジ博士課程を修了し帰国．長野県看護大学大学院 助教授，国立看護大学校 教授，日本看護協会勤務を経て2004年に看護ラボラトリーを開業し，代表となる（研修講師，コンサルタント）．専門は看護診断学．

おもな著書・訳書："看護師のための英会話ハンドブック"（共著，東京化学同人），"基本から見直す看護診断"（単著，医学芸術社），"アセスメント覚え書 ゴードン機能的健康パターンと看護診断"（訳，医学書院）

目　　次

はじめに：基本の基本 …………………………………………………… 1
ボディーランゲージ ……………………………………………………… 5

第 I 部　英文の書き方

Chapter 1　書き方の基本 …………………………………………… 9
Chapter 2　自己紹介書の書き方 ……………………… Track 1,2* … 11
Chapter 3　メールの書き方の基本 ………………………………… 13
Chapter 4　友人へのメールの書き方 ……………………………… 15
Chapter 5　まだ知らない人へのメールや手紙の書き方 ………… 20
　5・1　メールの書き方 ……………………………………………… 20
　5・2　手紙の書き方 ………………………………………………… 24
Chapter 6　就職に向けた自己アピールの書き方 ………………… 27
Chapter 7　英語での履歴書の書き方 ……………………………… 31

第 II 部　話し方・聞き方

Chapter 8　話し方・聞き方の基本 ………………………………… 41
　8・1　息継ぎ ………………………………………… Track 3 … 41
　8・2　イントネーション（抑揚）………………………………… 42
　8・3　話す速さ ……………………………………………………… 43

---

*　本書にはネイティブスピーカーにより録音された音声 CD が付録として付いています．Track 1〜26 は，その項の音声が CD に収録されていることを示しています．

Chapter 9　Please, Thank you, Excuse me の使い方 ………………………… 44
　9・1　"Please" の使い方 …………………………………… Track 4 … 44
　9・2　"Thank you" の使い方 ……………………………… Track 5 … 45
　9・3　"Excuse me" の使い方 ……………………………… Track 6 … 46
Chapter 10　挨　　拶 ………………………………………………… Track 7 … 47
Chapter 11　自然な英語での自己紹介 ………………………… Track 8, 9 … 49
Chapter 12　スモールトーク：好ましい質問と質問への答え方 ………… 51
　12・1　スモールトーク（スポーツ）…………………… Track 10 … 52
　12・2　スモールトーク（家族）………………………… Track 11 … 53
　12・3　スモールトーク（ペット）……………………… Track 12 … 54
　12・4　スモールトーク（旅行）………………………… Track 13 … 55
　12・5　スモールトーク（食べ物）……………………… Track 14 … 56
Chapter 13　ネイティブスピーカーの英語の発音 ………………………… 61
　13・1　言　　葉 ……………………………………… Track 15〜18 … 61
　13・2　二つ以上の言葉 ……………………………… Track 19〜21 … 62
　13・3　短　縮　形 ……………………………………… Track 22 … 64
Chapter 14　面　　接 ……………………………………………… Track 23, 24 … 66

第Ⅲ部　プレゼンテーションの上達法

Chapter 15　プレゼンテーションの上達法 ………………… Track 25, 26 … 71

付　　録

付録 A　薬学領域の科目名 ………………………………………………… 81
付録 B　薬学に関する職業 ………………………………………………… 82
付録 C　薬局・病院でよく使われる単語，頭字語，略語 ………………… 83
付録 D　薬局・病院でよく使われるラテン語由来の略語 ………………… 84
付録 E　短所を長所に変える表現（履歴書向け）………………………… 85

Eric's Tips

1. 会話は相手の目を見て大きな声で …………………………… 2
2. 適切な連絡手段を選択しよう ……………………………… 4
3. 不適切な笑いに注意 ………………………………………… 6
4. 件名は忘れずに ……………………………………………… 14
5. スペルに気をつけましょう ………………………………… 16
6. メールの返信（1）…………………………………………… 17
7. メールの返信（2）…………………………………………… 19
8. 目上の人へのメールで注意すること ……………………… 22
9. 大文字の使い方に注意 ……………………………………… 23
10. 就職活動中の服装：基本（1）……………………………… 26
11. 就職活動中の服装：基本（2）……………………………… 30
12. 就職活動中の服装：小物編 ………………………………… 32
13. 強気でいこう！ ……………………………………………… 38
14. 質問時のイントネーション ………………………………… 42
15. ドアを通るときのマナー …………………………………… 46
16. 質問の内容に注意 …………………………………………… 53
17. 自分で答えにくい質問は避けましょう …………………… 54
18. "hate" は使ってはダメ！ …………………………………… 55
19. 知っておきたい海外生活のマナーと表現 ………………… 57
20. 初心者は使わないほうがイイ ……………………………… 62
21. 聞き取れないときは丁寧に聞き返す ……………………… 64
22. 立ち振る舞いにも気をつけましょう ……………………… 72
23. くしゃみ，咳，あくび ……………………………………… 74

本文イラスト：望月さやか

はじめに：基本の基本
Before We Start

　プロらしい英語コミュニケーションとは，常識をわきまえた，知的で丁寧なコミュニケーションを意味します．英語を学習したり使ったりするときには，以下の1〜5を忘れないでおきましょう．

　1　"話し方で人となりがわかる"と言われます．丁寧で知的な英語を使う人は，良いイメージをもたれやすいものです．逆に，乱暴で不適切な英語を使う人は，悪いイメージをもたれてしまう可能性があります（図1）．このことは，本書全体を通して学習していただきたい重要なテーマです．

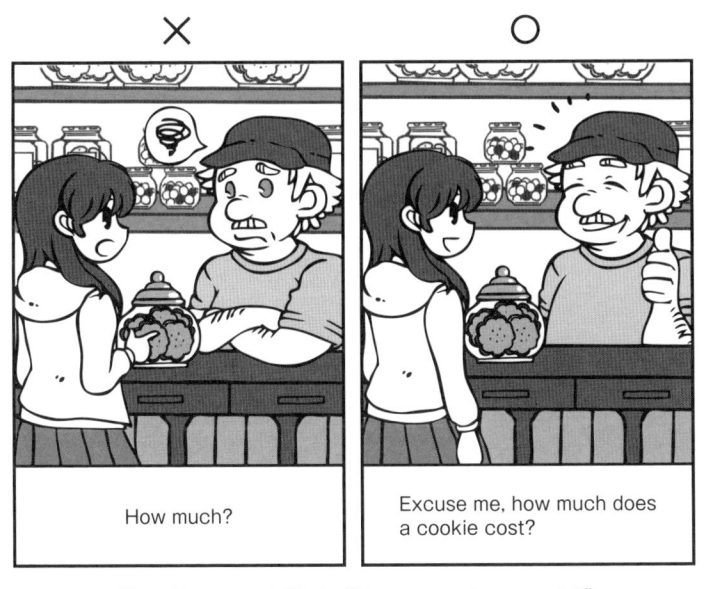

図1　"How much?" と "Excuse me, how much?"

2　英語と日本語には，綴り方と発音という点での大きな違いがあります．日本語の場合，母音の"あ，い，う，え，お"は文字どおりに発音します．日本人には当たりまえのことですが，英語を母語としている人（ネイティブスピーカー）が日本語を学習する際にはこれが大きな障壁になります．なぜでしょうか？　英語の場合，"a, e, i, o, u"を正確に綴ることは重要ですが，発音は常に文字どおりとは限らないからです（図2）．

たとえば，

(記述)　Today, I went shopping. Tomorrow, I will go to work.

と文字には書きますが，たいていのネイティブスピーカーは，

(発音)　Taday, I went shapping. Tamarrow, I will goda werk.

と発音します．この場合，"o"は常に"a"と発音したほうが自然な英語になります．多くの日本人がネイティブスピーカーの話を聞き取れない理由の一つがこれです．

ほかの例としては，

(記述)　Would you like something to eat?
(発音)　Woudja like somethin ta eat?

(記述)　I would like to study abroad in Boston.
(発音)　I'd like ta study abroad in Bastin.

(記述)　Can you give me a hand? I need your help.
(発音)　Kennya gimme a hand? I needjour help.

(記述)　She went to the store with him to buy some coffee.
(発音)　She wentta tha store withim ta buy sum caffee.

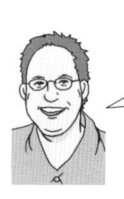

Eric's Tip 1　会話は相手の目を見て大きな声で

相手の目を見て大きな声で話しましょう．英語がいくら正確でも，目を見ずに小さな声で話したのでは，相手は理解してくれないことがあります．

以上はほんの一例ですが，本書ではほかにもさまざまな例を紹介します．

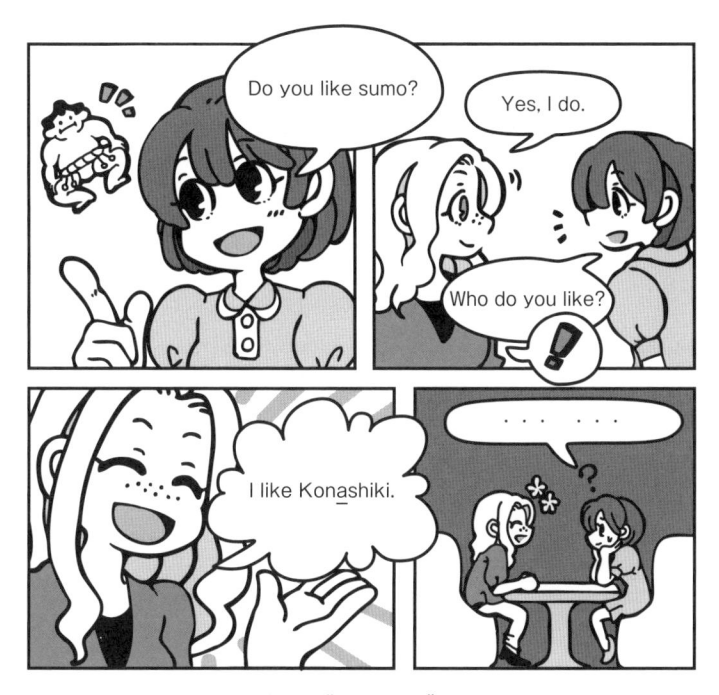

図2 "Konashiki"？

3　日本語と同様に英語でも，話をする相手との関係性をふまえることが重要です．親しい友人と英語で話をするときは，互いにカジュアルな英語を使います．けれども，親しくない人と話をするときには，丁寧な口調の英語を使います．

　話をする相手が男性か女性かはあまり重要ではありません．とは言っても，紳士ならば女性に対して礼儀正しく話をするのは当然のことです．日本語でもそうであるように，常識的な人は年長者には礼儀正しく丁寧に話をします．

4　日本語と同じく英語でも，言い回しが長くなればなるほど丁寧な表現になります．たとえば，誰かから何かをもらって"Thank you."と言う場合，

何通りもの表現が可能です．

　　・I sincerely appreciate your gift.
　　・Thank you for your present.
　　・Thanks for this.
　　・Thanks.

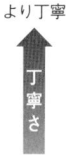

（より丁寧　↑　丁寧さ）

　最初の例文が最も長くて一番丁寧な言い回しです．"Thanks."だけでもマナー違反にはなりませんが，丁寧な口調とは言えません．カジュアルでくだけた言い回しです．

　また初対面の人への挨拶では，

　　・I am honored to finally meet you in person. I have heard so many good things about you.
　　・It is a pleasure to meet you.
　　・Nice to meet you.
　　・Nicetameecha.

（より丁寧　↑　丁寧さ）

　"Thanks."と同じく"Nice to meet you."もマナー違反ではありませんが，丁寧な言い回しではありません．言い回しが長いほど丁寧な表現になります．

5　最後に，英語と日本語にみられるプロらしいコミュニケーションの一番の違いですが，責任の所在にあるのではないかと思います．英語の場合，確実なコミュニケーションを図る責任は，話し手/書き手にあると考えられています．しかし日本語の場合は，聞き手/読み手に，伝達内容を把握する努力が期待されることが多いのではないでしょうか．

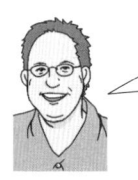

> **Eric's Tip 2　適切な連絡手段を選択しよう**
>
> 　会話はその重要性に応じて手段を選びましょう．質問や発言をするときは，対面＞手紙＞テレビ電話＞電話＞パソコンメール＞携帯メール＞SNS（フェイスブックなど）の順で使う手段を考えましょう．とても重要な内容は，メール（パソコンも携帯も）で伝えてはダメです．

ボディーランゲージ
Body Language

　最近の研究によると，人間のコミュニケーションの70％は身振りや表情によるものだそうです．自然な身振りや表情を活用すれば，コミュニケーションはスムーズにいくでしょう．逆に，自然な身振りや表情なしでは，コミュニケーションは阻害されるともいえます．ボディーランゲージにはよく気をつけて下さい．

　英語を長く教えるなかでよく目にするのは，話す際に身振りをまったく使わない人や，変わった身振りを使う人です．これでは自然な会話はできません．たとえば，"私は…"と自分について話す際に，鼻を指さしてはいけません．これは日本的な身振りです．英語を話しているときに自分を示すのであれば，胸を指さしましょう．

　以下に，プロらしい英語でのコミュニケーションに役立つ身振りを紹介します．会話中に出てくる数字の1から5は，図3のように指で示すと自然です．

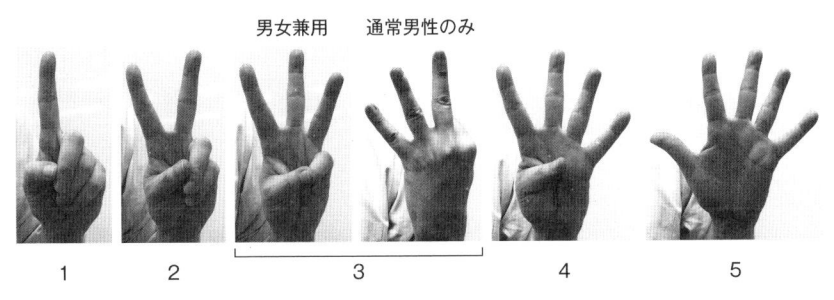

図3　ボディーランゲージ：英語の数字の表し方

　そのほか，よく使われる身振りを図4にあげます．

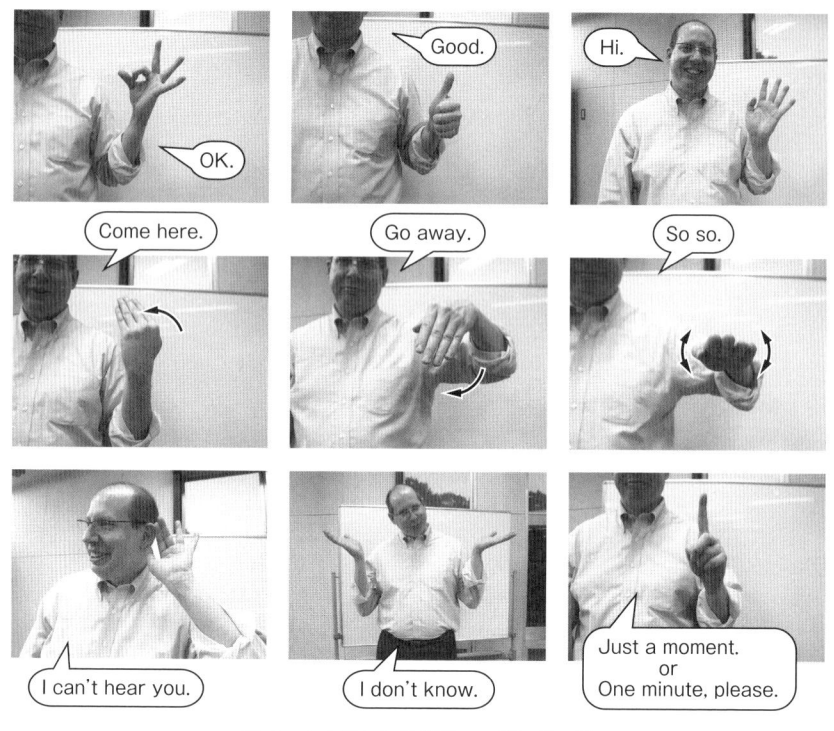

図4　よく使われるボディーランゲージ

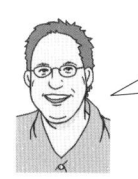

Eric's Tip 3　不適切な笑いに注意

不適切な笑いは避けましょう．（緊張のためか，自分の語学力に自信がないためか）笑いながら英語を話す日本人を多く見かけます．大切な話をするときは，けっして笑ってはいけません．誰かが真剣に話しかけてきたときも，絶対に笑ってはダメです．

I

英文の書き方

Writing Skills

東京化学同人
新刊とおすすめの書籍
Vol. 17

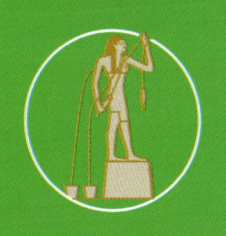

邦訳10年ぶりの改訂！　大学化学への道案内に最適

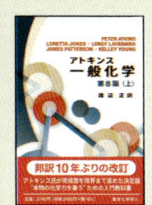

アトキンス 一般化学（上・下）
第8版

P. Atkins ほか著／渡辺 正訳

B5判　カラー　定価各3740円
上巻：320ページ　下巻：328ページ

"本物の化学力を養う"ための入門教科書

アトキンス氏が完成度を限界まで高めた決定版！大学化学への道案内に最適．高校化学の復習からはじまり，絶妙な全体構成で身近なものや現象にフォーカスしている．明快な図と写真，豊富な例題と復習問題付．

有機化学の基礎とともに生物学的経路への理解が深まる

マクマリー 有機化学
―生体反応へのアプローチ―　**第3版**

John McMurry 著

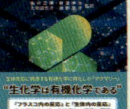

柴﨑正勝・岩澤伸治・大和田智彦・増野匡彦 監訳

B5変型判　カラー　960ページ　定価9790円

生命科学系の諸学科を学ぶ学生に役立つことを目標に書かれた有機化学の教科書最新改訂版．有機化学の基礎概念，基礎知識をきわめて簡明かつ完璧に記述するとともに，研究者が日常研究室内で行っている反応とわれわれの生体内の反応がいかに類似しているかを，多数の実例をあげて明確に説明している．

● 一般化学

- 教養の化学：暮らしのサイエンス　　定価 2640 円
- 教養の化学：生命・環境・エネルギー　定価 2970 円
- ブラックマン基礎化学　　　　　　　定価 3080 円
- 理工系のための一般化学　　　　　　定価 2750 円
- スミス基礎化学　　　　　　　　　　定価 2420 円

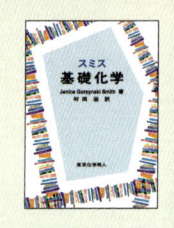

● 物理化学

- きちんと単位を書きましょう：国際単位系(SI)に基づいて　定価 1980 円
- 物理化学入門：基本の考え方を学ぶ　　定価 2530 円
- アトキンス物理化学要論（第 7 版）　　定価 6490 円
- アトキンス物理化学 上・下（第 10 版）　上巻定価 6270 円
  下巻定価 6380 円

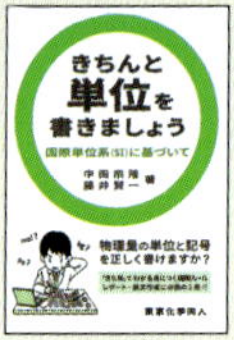

● 無機化学

- シュライバー・アトキンス無機化学（第 6 版）上・下　定価各 7150 円
- 基礎講義 無機化学　　　　　　　　　定価 2860 円

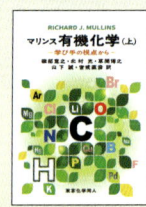

● 有機化学

- マクマリー有機化学概説（第 7 版）　　定価 5720 円
- マリンス有機化学　上・下　　　　　　定価各 7260 円
- クライン有機化学　上・下　　　　　　定価各 6710 円
- ラウドン有機化学　上・下　　　　　　定価各 7040 円
- ブラウン有機化学　上・下　　　　　　定価各 6930 円
- 有機合成のための新触媒反応 101　　　定価 4620 円
- 構造有機化学：基礎から物性へのアプローチまで　定価 5280 円
- スミス基礎有機化学　　　　　　　　　定価 2640 円

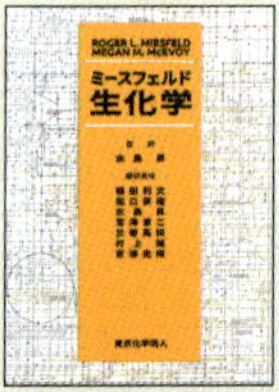

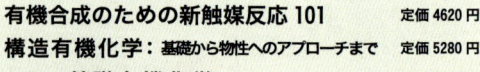

● 生化学・細胞生物学

- スミス基礎生化学　　　　　　　　　　定価 2640 円
- 相分離生物学　　　　　　　　　　　　定価 3520 円
- ヴォート基礎生化学（第 5 版）　　　　定価 8360 円
- ミースフェルド生化学　　　　　　　　定価 8690 円
- 分子細胞生物学（第 9 版）　　　　　　定価 9570 円

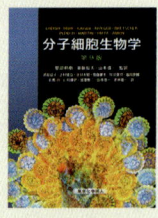

お問い合わせ info@tkd-pbl.com　　定価は 10 % 税込

● 生物学

モリス生物学：生命のしくみ	定価 9900 円
スター生物学（第6版）	定価 3410 円
初歩から学ぶ ヒトの生物学	定価 2970 円

● 基礎講義シリーズ（講義動画付）
アクティブラーニングにも対応

基礎講義 遺伝子工学 I・II	定価各 2750 円
基礎講義 分子生物学	定価 2860 円
基礎講義 生化学	定価 3080 円
基礎講義 生物学	定価 2420 円
基礎講義 物理学	定価 2420 円
基礎講義 天然物医薬品化学	定価 3740 円

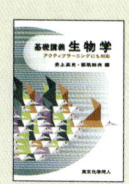

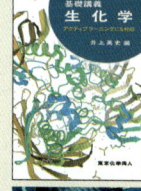

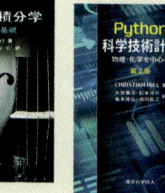

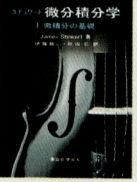

● 数 学

スチュワート微分積分学 I～III（原著第8版）

I．微積分の基礎	定価 4290 円
II．微積分の応用	定価 4290 円
III．多変数関数の微分積分	定価 4290 円

● コンピューター・情報科学

ダイテル Python プログラミング 　基礎からデータ分析・機械学習まで	定価 5280 円
Python 科学技術計算 物理・化学を中心に（第2版）	定価 5720 円
Python, TensorFlow で実践する 深層学習入門 　しくみの理解と応用	定価 3960 円
R で基礎から学ぶ 統計学	定価 4180 円

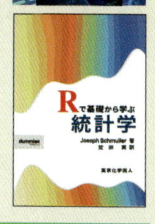

現代化学　CHEMISTRY TODAY

広い視野と教養を培う月刊誌
毎月18日発売　定価 1100 円

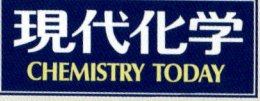

◆ 最前線の研究動向をいち早く紹介
◆ 第一線の研究者自身による解説やインタビュー
◆ 理解を促し考え方を学ぶ基礎講座
◆ 科学の素養が身につく教養満載

カラーの図や写真多数

電子版あります！

定期購読しませんか？
定期購読がとってもお得です!!
お申込みはこちら→

購読期間（冊数：定価）	冊子版（送料無料）
6カ月（6冊：~~6,600円~~） ▶	4,600 円（1冊あたり767円）
1カ年（12冊：~~13,200円~~） ▶	8,700 円（1冊あたり725円）
2カ年（24冊：~~26,400円~~） ▶	15,800 円（1冊あたり658円）

おすすめの書籍

女性が科学の扉を開くとき
偏見と差別に対峙した六〇年
NSF（米国国立科学財団）長官を務めた科学者が語る

リタ・コルウェル, シャロン・バーチュ・マグレイン 著
大隅典子 監訳／古川奈々子 訳／定価 3520 円

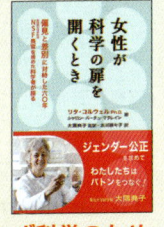

科学界の差別と向き合った体験をとおして，男女問わず科学のために何ができるかを呼びかける．科学への情熱が眩しい一冊．

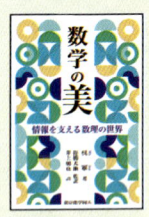

元 Google 開発者が語る，簡潔を是とする思考法
数学の美　情報を支える数理の世界

呉　軍 著／持橋大地 監訳／井上朋生 訳／定価 3960 円

Google 創業期から日中韓三ヵ国語の自然言語処理研究を主導した著者が，自身の専門である自然言語処理や情報検索を中心に，情報革新を生み出した数学について語る．開発者たちの素顔や思考法とともに紹介．

月刊誌【現代化学】の対談連載より書籍化 第1弾
桝 太一が聞く 科学の伝え方

桝　太一 著／定価 1320 円

サイエンスコミュニケーションとは何か？ どんな解決すべき課題があるのか？ 桝先生と一緒に答えを探してみませんか？

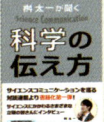

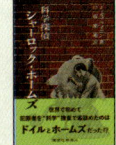

科学探偵 シャーロック・ホームズ

J. オブライエン 著・日暮雅通 訳／定価 3080 円

世界で初めて犯人を科学捜査で追い詰めた男の物語．シャーロッキアンな科学の専門家が科学をキーワードにホームズの物語を読み解く．

新版 鳥はなぜ集まる？ 群れの行動生態学
科学のとびら 65

上田恵介 著／定価 1980 円

臨機応変に維持される鳥の群れの仕組みを，社会生物学の知見から鳥類学者が柔らかい語り口でひもとくよみもの．

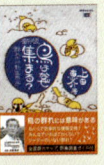

Chapter 1

書き方の基本
Writing Basics

　プライベートでも仕事でも，適切に英文を書くことは，21世紀における最も重要なコミュニケーションスキルの一つです．なお，フェイスブックなどへの投稿は，仕事で手紙を書く場合とは要領が異なります．

■ 基本の書き方

　何か文章を書く際は"The Rule of Three－Essay"（文書の三部構成）を使います．すなわち，

- ①　序　論（Introduction）
- ②　本　論（Body）
- ③　結　論（Conclusion）

の三つが必要です．プロらしく文章を書くためには，この基本原則を覚えておきましょう（図5）．

　メールや手紙は"The Rule of Three－Letter"（手紙の三部構成）を使い，

- ①　書き出しの挨拶（First greeting）
- ②　内　容（Message）
- ③　結びの挨拶（Final greeting）

の順番で書きます．

Essay（文書），Sentence（文）		
Introduction （序　論）	Body （本　論）	Conclusion （結　論）
E-mail（メール），Letter（手紙）		
First greeting （書き出しの挨拶）	Message （内　容）	Final greeting （結びの挨拶）

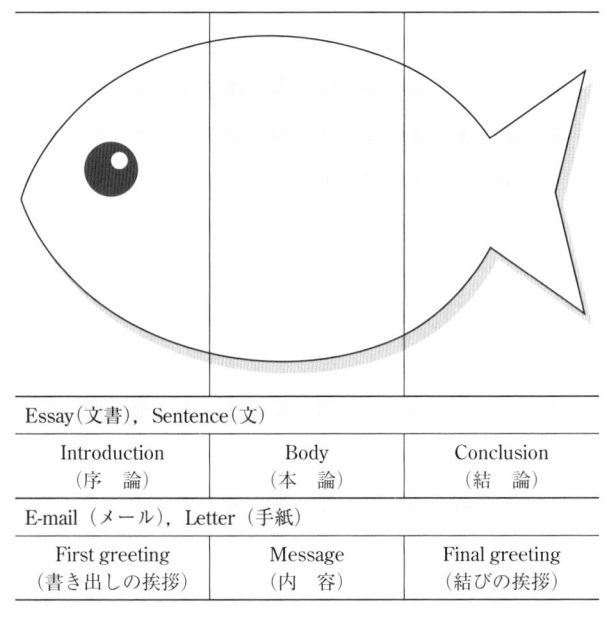

図 5　文書の三部構成

　一般的な英文は，"The Rule of Three-Sentence"（文の三部構成）に従います．つまり英語の文章には，

　　1　主　語（Subject）
　　2　述　語（Verb）
　　3　目的語（Object）

が含まれます．一部分でも抜けてしまうと，あなたが伝えたいことが読み手に伝わらなくなってしまいます．
　英語を書く際にはこれらの原則に従いましょう．

Chapter 2

自己紹介書の書き方
Writing Self-introductions

就職活動中，英語で書いた自己紹介書の提出を求められるかもしれません．以下に簡単で効果的な自己紹介書の書き方の例をあげます．

Example 1

My name is Genki Mukaide[*1] and I am a 5th-year student pharmacist at Tokyo College of Pharmacy. My favorite subject is biochemistry and I play the violin in the school orchestra. In the future, I hope to work in a hospital.

*1 英語で氏名を書くときは，名前が先で苗字は後です．そうしないと，日本人でない人は，名前と苗字を勘違いしてしまいます．

Example 2

I am Atsushi Yamada and I am a 6th-year student pharmacist at Osaka College of Pharmacy. My favorite subject is immunology and I am a runner on the track team. In the future, I will work as a CRA in an international pharmaceutical company.

上記の 2 例はいずれも "The Rule of Three－Sentence"（文の三部構成）に従って，主語・述語・目的語が含まれています．現在（自分は誰で何が好きか）と将来（どのような仕事に就きたいか）のバランスもとれています．簡単です

が，とても良い自己紹介書の書き方です．

▶ Checklist ☑
- ☐ 氏 名（Full name）
- ☐ 学 年（Year of study）
- ☐ 得意な科目（Favorite subject）
- ☐ 趣味/部活動（Hobby/School activity）
- ☐ 希望する仕事（Desired job）

Useful Expressions

1) 薬学生：student pharmacist, pharmacy student（student pharmacist のほうが，pharmacy student よりもプロらしい表現です．）
2) 1st-, 2nd-, 3rd-, 4th-, 5th-, または 6th-year[*2] student（それぞれ1年生，2年生，3年生，4年生，5年生，6年生の表現方法です．）

   [*2] 大学生の場合，"grade" は用いません．"grade" は小学生，中学生，高校生の場合に使用します．

3) 代表的な科目とその英語は，付録A（p.81）を参照．
4) 代表的な仕事（職種）とその英語は，付録B（p.82）を参照．

Chapter 3

メールの書き方の基本
E-mail Writing Basics

どのようなメールにも以下の[1]〜[7]を含め，この順番で構成するのが基本です．

[1] あなたの名前（メールソフトの設定を必ずローマ字にしておくこと）と返信先のメールアドレス
[2] 件 名：送るメールの目的・用件を端的に表現しましょう．
[3] 宛 名：送信先の人の名前を書きます．

> **Examples 1**
>
> Dear Eric,
> Dear Mr. Skier,
> Dear Ms. Fukutomi,
> Dear Dr. Hara,

友人へのメールであれば，かしこまらず，ファーストネームを使って"Hi Eric,"や"Hello Steve,"のように書きましょう．

[4] 書き出しの挨拶 ◁1◁

> **Examples 2**
>
> Thank you for your e-mail the other day.
> How are you? I hope everything is fine.
> The weather is very nice recently. Have you enjoyed it?
> Recently many people have the flu. I hope you are well.

5　メールの内容・目的の端的な説明

> **Examples 3**
>
> By the way (BTW), here is this week's homework.
> By the way, here is the information you asked for.

6　結びの挨拶

> **Examples 4**
>
> Thank you for your time.
> Thank you for your help.
> I hope this_____.
> (_____には is useful, is all right, will help などが入ります)
> Appreciatively,
> Best regards,
> Respectfully,

7　署　名：本文の最後に自分の名前と連絡先などの重要な情報を署名欄に書きます．

Name：
Student year：
Department/lab name：
University name：
　(phone number, Skype address, and mailing address)

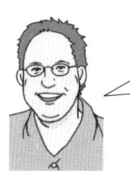

Eric's Tip 4　件名は忘れずに

メールには"件名（subject）"を必ずつけること．受け取る人はたくさんのメールを読まなければなりません．"件名"のないメールは重要ではないと思われてしまう恐れがあります．

Chapter 4

友人へのメールの書き方
Writing E-mail to a Friend

本章では友人に向けたメールの書き方を学びます.まずは下記の例文1から見ていきましょう.

<例文 1>

From: Ken Watanabe <kenw@kyushu.xxx.com>
To: Chris Myer <chris@houston.xxx.com>
Cc:
Subject: Trip to Houston

Hello Chris,[*1]

How are you? I hope you are well. I am OK, but I am busy with my studies. I am studying hard to pass my big test to become a pharmacist. How about you? How are your studies? ①

By the way, I will be going to Houston next month. It would be great to see you. I hope we can meet and have some Texas BBQ. ②

I look forward to hearing from you, ③
Ken

------------------------------------[*2]
Ken Watanabe
5th-year student pharmacist
Microbiology Laboratory
Kyushu College of Pharmaceutical Science
kenw@kyushu.xxx.com
----

*1 親しい友人にはファーストネームを使います．まだよく知らない人に，ファーストネームを使ってはいけません．
*2 署名の上下にラインを入れたほうが，プロらしいメールに見えますし，署名を判別しやすくなります．ラインは署名内容よりも少しだけ長めにします．

例文 1 のメール文は下記のように構成されています．Chapter 1 で学んだ基本 "文章の三部構成" を忠実に守っていますね．

1. "書き出しの挨拶" に相当する部分

How are you? I hope you are well. I am OK, but I am busy with my studies. I am studying hard to pass my big test to become a pharmacist. How about you? How are your studies?

2. "内容" に相当する部分

By the way, I will be going to Houston next month. It would be great to see you. I hope we can meet and have some Texas BBQ.

3. "結びの挨拶" に相当する部分

I look forward to hearing from you,

次ページでもう一つ例をみてみましょう．

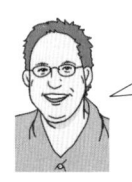

Eric's Tip 5　スペルに気をつけましょう

スペルに気をつけましょう．スペルに自信がなく，メールにスペルチェック機能がない場合は，まず MS Word などのチェック機能のついたワープロソフト上で文章を作成し，スペルをチェックしてから，メールにコピー＆ペーストしましょう．

Chapter 4 友人へのメールの書き方

<例文 2>

From: Ai Kusanagi <akusanagi@jcop.xxx.com>
To: Jennifer Smith <jennifer@america.xxx.com>
Cc:
Subject: Japan Visit

Hi Jennifer,

Long time, no hear!*3 I hope you and your loved ones are all OK. My family and I are fine. We are all busy with life in general. ⟨1⟩

By the way, I heard you will come to Japan next year. Is that true? If so, it would be great to see you.
If possible, please let me know your schedule. ⟨2⟩

Looking forward to hearing from you, ⟨3⟩
Ai

Ai Kusanagi
6th-year student pharmacist
Biochemistry Laboratory
Japan College of Pharmacy
akusanagi@jcop.xxx.com
----

*3 直接会って話をしているときの"久しぶり"は"Long time, no see."と言いますが,メールでは"Long time, no hear."となります.

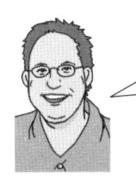

Eric's Tip 6 メールの返信（1）

メールは 24 時間以内に返信しましょう．メールを送る人はあなたからの返信がすぐに来ることを期待しています．

例文1，2は，どちらも友人に当てたメールです．バランスがよくとれています．

まず挨拶を"Hello,"や"Hi,"で始めて，"Long time, no hear."などを続け，相手や家族についての近況を尋ねます．("Long time, no hear."は，間隔が1週間以上空いた場合にだけ用います．）つづいて自分の近況を知らせます．

つぎに内容ですが，たいていは"By the way,"で始めます．最後に，結びの挨拶を書きます．友人への丁寧で適切なメールになっています．

▶ Checklist ☑

- ☐ 友人の氏名（Friend's name）
- ☐ 書き出しの挨拶（First greeting）
- ☐ 内　容（Letter/E-mail message）
- ☐ 結びの挨拶（Final greeting）
- ☐ 自分の名前（友人にはファーストネームが適切）（Your name）

Useful Expressions

1) こんにちは　　　Hello　　　より丁寧
　　　　　　　　　Hi
　　　　　　　　　Hey
　　　　　　　　　Yo

2) お元気ですか？　　Long time, no hear.　　より丁寧
　　　　　　　　　　How are you?
　　　　　　　　　　What's up?
　　　　　　　　　　Whassup?

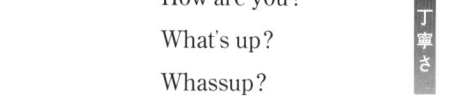

3) あなたとご家族のご健康をお祈りいたします．
　　　I hope you and your loved ones are well.　　より丁寧
　　　I hope you and your family are well.
　　　I hope you are well.

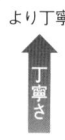

4) 自分の近況を伝える表現

　　I am great! / Life is good! / Everything is fine here.
　　I am fine. / I am well. / I am OK. / I am doing OK.
　　I am hanging in there. / I am not doing so well. / Life is so-so.
　　Actually, I am not well.

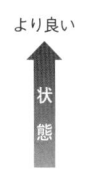

より良い　↑　状態

手紙の冒頭で不幸な近況を友人に知らせるのは，マナーとしてあまり好ましいものではありません．最初は良い（明るい）ことを書いてから，問題や不幸を知らせましょう．

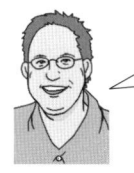

> **Eric's Tip 7　メールの返信（2）**
> 　文法の間違いに気をつけましょう．**Eric's Tip 5**のコツと同様，MS Wordなどのチェック機能のついたワープロソフトを用いるのもよいでしょう．完全に修正はできませんが，まったくしないよりもずっとましです．

Chapter 5

まだ知らない人への
メールや手紙の書き方

Writing E-mail or Letters to Someone for the First Time

　本章では，まだ連絡をとったことのない人に向けた丁寧なメール，手紙の書き方を学びます．

5・1　メールの書き方

＜例文 1＞

From：Ayako Sato <asato@ejcps.xxx.com>
To：<Moreau@america.xxx.com>
Cc：
Subject：Study Abroad Question

Dear Ms. Moreau,[*1, *2]

My name is Ayako Sato. I am writing to ask you some questions about your study abroad program.[*3, *4] ｝ 1

First, will I be able to stay on campus? Second, what do you recommend I bring with me for my studies? Lastly, will there be a chance to go sightseeing on the weekends? ｝ 2

I look forward to your reply,[*5] ｝ 3
Ayako[*6]

Ayako Sato
6th-year student pharmacist
Immunology Laboratory
East Japan College of Pharmaceutical Science
asato@ejcps.xxx.com
----

*1 冒頭の挨拶のマナーとして"Dear"を使います．
*2 "Mr." または "Ms." をフルネームの前につけます．一般的に，Mrs. は使いません．相手が Ph.D. または M.D. を取得している場合は，"Dr." をつけましょう．わかっていれば，相手の肩書きを書きます．
*3 初めて手紙を出すときは常に自己紹介から始めます．
*4 自分自身のこと，および，このメールを出す理由について説明を加えます．
*5 相手からの連絡がほしい場合，この文を加えることはとても重要です．
*6 フォーマルな手紙を書く際には，改行して名前を書きます．親しくなりたければ，ファーストネームだけにします．よりプロらしくするならば，フルネーム（氏名）を書きます．

▶ Checklist ☑

☐ 挨　拶（Greeting）
☐ 相手の氏名（Name）
☐ 簡単な自己紹介（Introduce yourself briefly）
☐ 手紙を書いている理由（Explain why you are contacting the person）
☐ 手紙/メールの内容（Letter/E-mail message）
☐ 結びの挨拶（Final greeting）
☐ 自分の名前（氏名）（Your name）

Useful Expressions

1) 本文で，嬉しい・悲しい・怒りなどの，自分の本当の気持ちを表現しているときに用いる結びの挨拶

　　　　Yours sincerely,　　↑ より丁寧
　　　　Sincerely yours,　　丁寧さ

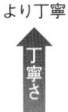

2）相手に何かをお願いする場合，何かしてくれた場合に使う表現

    Thank you for your time, より丁寧

    Appreciatively yours,

    Gratefully yours,   丁寧さ

    Yours gratefully,

    Thank you,

    Thanks,

3）返信するときや何か情報を伝えるときに使う表現
（実際にはあまり使いません）

    Best regards,

    Regards,

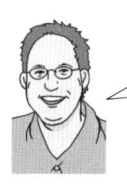

Eric's Tip 8　目上の人へのメールで注意すること

"Thank you in advance" は目下の人に使う表現なので，目上の人に送るメールや手紙では使ってはいけません．

<例文 2>

From: Kazuhiro Suzuki <kazuhiros@wjcp.xxx.com>
To: <Aramaki@tupls.xxx.com>
Cc:
Subject: About Your Lab

Dear Prof. Aramaki,

My name is Kazuhiro Suzuki and I am a 4th-year student pharmacist. ⟩①

I am interested in studying in your lab. Could you tell me what I will learn if I join your laboratory? When do you have your seminar? Will there be a chance to study abroad? ⟩②

Yours appreciatively, ⟩③
Kazuhiro

Kazuhiro Suzuki
4th-year student pharmacist
Western Japan College of Pharmacy
kazuhiros@wjcp.xxx.com

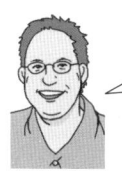

Eric's Tip 9　大文字の使い方に注意

大文字だけでメールを書くのはやめましょう．たとえば，NICE TO MEET YOU なんて書くと，機嫌が悪くて怒鳴っているように受け取られる可能性があります．ただし，お祝いの CONGRATULATIONS！ HAPPY BIRTHDAY！ などは例外です．

5・2 手紙の書き方

<例文 3>

> 123 ABC Road
> Tokyo, Japan, 165-0023*7
>
> November 30, 2012*8

Ms. Lisa Jones*9
Human Resources Director*10
XYZ Pharmaceutical Company
2345 Drug Lane
Los Angeles, CA. 93820-0045*11

Dear Ms. Jones： *12

Hello, my name is Hanako Suzuki and I am a 6th-year student pharmacist in Japan.*13

From next year I will start my doctoral studies and conduct research into the development of cancer drugs from natural products. After my studies are finished, I hope to study abroad and continue to do research.*14

While it is early, I am interested in possibly working for your company in the future. Is there any advice you can give me that would help me achieve this goal?

I look forward to hearing from you.*15

Sincerely yours,*16

Hanako*17

---

*7 返信がほしい場合は，ここに自分の住所を書きます．
*8 日付．ここに示したのは米国式です．英国式では日/月/年で表します．
*9 "Mr." または "Ms." をフルネームの前につけます．相手が Ph.D. または M.D. を取得している場合は，"Dr." をつけます．
*10 わかっていれば，相手の肩書きを書きます．

* 11　ここに自分が連絡をとりたい相手の住所を書きます.
* 12　個人的な手紙の場合は相手の名前の後にコンマ (,) を使いますが, ビジネスレターではコロン (:) を使います.
* 13　初めて手紙を出すときは常に自己紹介から始めます.
* 14　自分自身のこと, または, この手紙を書いている理由について説明を加えます.
* 15　結びの挨拶の1行目. 相手からの返信がほしい場合, この文を加えることはとても重要です.
* 16　忘れずに結びの挨拶文を書きます.
* 17　最後に署名します.(ファーストネームだけでもフルネームでも OK です.)

＜例文 4＞

9876 XYZ Avenue
Osaka, Japan, 456-0099

December 1, 2012

Human Resources Department [18]
Swiss Pharmaceutical Corporation
18 Drug Road
Geneva, Switzerland 54-98-09

To whom it may concern: [19]

My name is Taro Harada and I am a 3rd-year student pharmacist at the Tokyo College of Pharmacy. After speaking to my adviser, I though I would write to ask you about your company.

I am interested in doing an internship in your company. In the future, I hope to work in an international pharmaceutical company and would love to meet some of your employees to learn about the various positions in your company.

If it is possible for me to do an internship, please let me know when and what I need to do to participate in this program.

Thank you for your time and I look forward to hearing from you.

Yours appreciatively,

Taro

＊18 会社あてに出す場合で，担当者名がわからないときは，部署名または役職名（たとえば Human Resources Director など）を書きます．

＊19 相手の氏名がわからない場合であっても，ここには何か必ず書かなくてはいけません．"To whom it may concern:" とするのが，礼儀正しく，プロらしい書き方です．

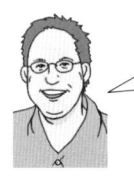

Eric's Tip 10　就職活動中の服装: 基本 (1)
　日本では就職活動中の個性のない"リクルートスーツ"は当たり前ですが，海外にはこのような文化はありません．センスのよいスーツ（黒はダメ），ネクタイ，シャツ，ベルト，靴を選びましょう．

Chapter 6

就職に向けた自己アピールの書き方
Writing about Yourself when Job-hunting

　製薬会社の多くが英語のできる人を採用したいと考えるようになってきました．就職活動中には，自分についてのエッセイが課されることもあります．自分自身についての書き方は，日本語と英語では異なる点が多くあります．

　自分について書く際，三部構成の原則に従いましょう．エッセイには，序論，本論，結論の三つを含めます．以下に例をあげます．

＜例　文＞

My name is Keisuke Higashi. I am the middle child and have two sisters*1. I have been studying the pharmaceutical sciences*2 and my favorite subject has been organic chemistry. I have also been active in the kendo club and was the leader of the club when I was a 3rd-year student.*3

I hope to get a job as a clinical research associate (CRA) as I like meeting new people and have good coordinating skills. Your company interests me as it is a leader in various fields and develops drugs that help many people. I also understand that this is an international company and my experience living abroad may be very useful in such a work environment.

In conclusion, I look forward to working in your company in the future. I hope to have the opportunity to show you my talents and help your company.

Thank you for your time,

Keisuke Higashi

*1 彼は三人兄弟の真ん中で，姉と妹がいると伝えています．家族内の続柄は図6のように表現します．
*2 "pharmaceutical sciences" が "pharmacy" よりもプロらしい表現です．このようなエッセイでは "pharmaceutical sciences" を使います．
*3 できれば部活動について書きましょう．大学の部活動に参加していない人は，何も書く必要はありません．何かアルバイトをしていれば，それを書いてもよいでしょう．

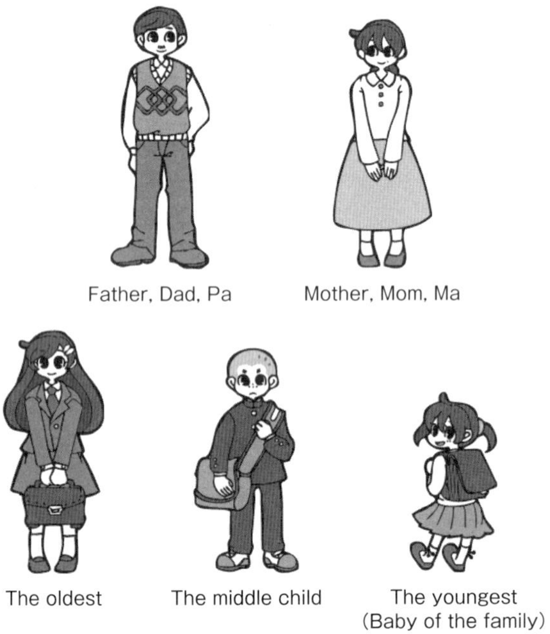

Father, Dad, Pa　　Mother, Mom, Ma

The oldest　　The middle child　　The youngest
(Baby of the family)

図6　家族内の続柄を示す英語

Chapter 6 就職に向けた自己アピールの書き方

▶ Checklist ☑

- ☐ 自己紹介（Introduce yourself）
- ☐ 家族についての簡単な紹介（Talk briefly about your family）
- ☐ 得意科目や研究の説明
  （Talk about your studies and favorite subject）
- ☐ 部活動やアルバイトについての説明
  （Talk about your club activities and part-time job）
- ☐ どのような仕事をしたいのかの説明，具体的に
  （Explain what kind of job you want in the company － be specific！）
- ☐ あれば，留学経験，海外での研修経験，海外でのホームステイ経験など
  （If possible, talk about your study abroad experience, home stay, etc...）
- ☐ 会社にどのように貢献したいのかの意思
  （Say something about how you want to contribute to the company）
- ☐ 結びの挨拶（Final greeting）

チェックリストに沿って書き進める際，自分の弱点やマイナスなイメージにつながるようなことを書いてはいけません．常にポジティブに！

Examples

①ネガティブ：My TOEIC score is 360.
　　　　　　　↓
　ポジティブ：I'm currently studying English very hard to improve my TOEIC score.

②ネガティブ：I haven't done much lab work.
　　　　　　　↓
　ポジティブ：I had good marks for all of my lab practices.

Useful Expressions

1) 好きな科目，得意な科目を伝える表現

   I have been studying the pharmaceutical sciences and my favorite subject has been _____ 〔付録A（p.81）参照〕.

2) 就きたい職種を伝えるときの表現

   I hope to get a job as a _____ 〔付録B（p.82）参照〕.

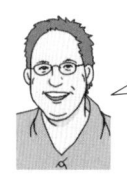

> **Eric's Tip 11　就職活動中の服装：基本（2）**
>
> 　自分の良さが引き立つような個性あるスタイルを見つけましょう．ヘアスタイルやメガネで工夫できます．他の人から際立つ必要はありませんが，印象に残る違いを出すことが重要です．
>
> 　男性の場合，白色のボタンダウン襟でない長袖シャツが最もフォーマルです．色ならば次に青系色です．ボタンダウン襟のシャツはカジュアルな服装なのでダメです．

Chapter 7

英語での履歴書の書き方
Writing a Resume in English

最近は，就職を目指す学生に英語の履歴書を提出させる企業もあります．英語の履歴書は日本語の履歴書とはずいぶんと異なります．たとえば，英語の履歴書には次のような資料や情報は不要です．

- 顔写真（A picture）
- 性別（Gender）
- 生年月日や年齢（Your birthday or age）
- 結婚しているかどうか（Any mention of being married or not）
- 通学・卒業した小学校，中学校，高校（No mention of elementary, junior high, or high school）

一般的に，英語の履歴書には以下の1〜6が必要です．

1. 希望する仕事：会社の中の具体的にどの職種に就きたいのか（An objective − what position in particular are you seeking in the company?）
2. 教育歴（Your education background）：
   最終学歴．たとえば，大学，大学院など
3. 職　歴（Your work experience）：
   特に目指している仕事に関係しているもの
4. 特　技：パソコン，外国語，など（Your skills: computer, language, etc...）
5. 免　許：薬剤師，自動車運転免許証，など（Licenses: pharmacist, driver's, etc...）
6. その他（Other）：他の応募者よりも自分を目立たせる事柄

何度も言いますが，自分自身についてネガティブなことを書いてはいけません．自分は何ができるのか，何が得意なのか，ポジティブなことだけを書きましょう〔付録E（p.85）参照〕．

つぎに一般的な履歴書の例を二つ紹介します（p.33〜38）．

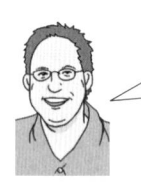

Eric's Tip 12　就職活動中の服装：小物編

　色の統一：身につける革製品（腕時計のベルト，鞄，靴，財布，ベルト）の色を揃えましょう．茶色の靴を履いて黒のベルトはカッコ悪い！

　靴下：濃い色のズボンや靴を履いたら，必ず靴下も濃い色で．スーツのときに，白い靴下は履かないこと！

　鞄：ショルダーバックは女性用です．男性が持っていると変な誤解をされる恐れがあります．書類，パソコン，財布などを入れるのは，ブリーフケースかメッセンジャーバッグにしましょう．鞄は2色（黒と茶色）を持っていると便利です．

　腕時計：男性諸君，シンプルで良い手巻きか自動巻きの時計を身につけましょう．ブラックタイ＆タキシードで出席するような場所に行く際には，革ベルトの時計をしましょう．女性ならば，シンプルなクォーツ時計がおススメです．

<履歴書の例 1>

CHIHIRO HARA

8-31-15 Nohara Yashio-ku, Tokyo 148-0210, Japan
Tel: 090-XXXX-YYYY
E-mail: hara-c_840@ZZZZ-u.ac.jp

Objective

To secure a supply chain position that will allow me to utilize my pharmaceutical knowledge and skills, and also allow me to grow and advance my business judgment skills within the organization.

Education

April, 2006 –
March, 2012
Yashio University of Pharmacy and Life Sciences, Yashio-ku, Tokyo

Bachelor of Science, Pharmacy
Lab Name: Medicinal Chemistry
Professor Name: Professor Kaoru Sumita
Graduation Thesis:
Research for Synthesis of Biologically Active Agents:
 Myxopyronin and Cyclosporine

Thesis details:
I did research on the synthesis of myxopyronin, an anti-bacterial product, and cyclosporine, an immunosuppressive product, as biologically active agents. Myxopyronin is expected to have effective anti-bacterial activity. However the lipid solubility prevents the drug discovery research. Therefore I undertook the research to make some derivatives that increase activity. Cyclosporine is a medicine used as an immunosuppressive drug. Currently, it is thought to have other effective actions. Therefore, I undertook this research to make some derivatives and to

examine the biological activities.

Lab activities consisted of:
- Every Monday: Graduation thesis seminar
This is a seminar where one person in charge of the day introduces a paper — it has included reading some studies, making a resume, and learning how to make presentations.
- Every Saturday: Organic synthesis seminars
This is a seminar where we learned about organic reaction mechanisms through the study of total synthesis.

May, 2010− July, 2010	Hospital practice at Jikei University Daisan Hospital, Komae-shi, Tokyo Activities included: Learning about the duties of a hospital pharmacist: filling prescriptions, dispensing injection drugs, drug administration guidance, and in-patient pharmaceutical service. I also learned about the duties of other health care professions such as: doctors, nurses, dietitians, radiation technologists, and laboratory technicians.
September, 2010− December, 2010	Community pharmacy practice at Aoba Pharmacy, Yakuju, Hino-shi, Tokyo Activities included: Learning about the duties of a community pharmacy pharmacist. In particular, how to fill a prescription, compounding, drug administration guidance, home medical care, and medical security systems.

Work Experience

May, 2010− March, 2011	**Izumi Pharmacy**, Setagaya-ku, Tokyo Duties included: Working as a general office clerk. I was typing prescriptions and did some accounting according to

the medical or social insurance schemes. In addition, I helped prepared drugs as a pharmacist assistant.

April, 2007– **Chiyoda-tutoring**, Chiyoda-ku, Tokyo
March, 2010 Duties included: Tutoring junior high school and high school students in English, mathematics, chemistry, physics, and biology to prepare students for high school or university entrance examinations.

Computer Skills
MS Word, Excel, Power Point, Chem Draw, and ISIS Draw

Language Skills
Japanese: Native speaker
English: Scored 700 on the TOEIC (June, 2010)

Licenses

June, 2007 First aromatherapy class
Took the license by self-study. This license is the first step to becoming an aromatherapy specialist. This also including learning how aromatherapy can help in healthcare.

August, 2007 Japanese driver's license

Other
Attendend IISIA preparatory school to learn information literacy (2011)
Member of Tahitian Dancing Society (2007–2009)
Studied English at LSI, Auckland, New Zealand for one month (August 2006)
Have traveled to more than 10 countries over the last five years.

<履歴書の例 2>

HIDEKI SUZUKI

16-330 Minami Igusa-shi, Kumamoto 869-8869, Japan
Tel: 090-XXXX-YYYY
E-mail: Suzuki_h_551@pharm_ZZZZ-u.ac.jp

Objective

I hope to get a position in an international pharmaceutical company working as a clinical research coordinator as I am very interested in helping with the development of new drug therapies.

Education

April, 2007-   **Kumamoto School of Pharmacy, Kumamoto, Japan**
March, 2013   Bachelor of Science, Pharmacy
　　　　　　　Lab Name: Drug Delivery Systems
　　　　　　　Professor Name: Professor Toshio Hirano
　　　　　　　Graduation Thesis:
　　　　　　　Research for Development of siRNA Targeting *bcl-2* as an Anti-cancer Active Agent
　　　　　　　Thesis details:
　　　　　　　I did research on a gene therapy for treating cancer by RNA interference. I synthesized siRNA, which knocked down *bcl-2*, an anti-apoptosis gene. The injection of the siRNA to Bcl-2 over-expression HL-60 cells efficiently led to apoptosis in those cells. This result suggests that the decrease in the Bcl-2 protein causes cancer cell death. Thus, siRNA may be a new type of anti-cancer drug.
　　　　　　　Lab activities consisted of:
　　　　　　　・Every Saturday: Graduation thesis seminar
　　　　　　　　　　　　　We did a journal club and had to present papers (in English) to the rest of the members of the laboratory. This

	helped me improve my English, presentation skills, and writing skills. ・Every Tuesday: Reading circle This was a seminar where one person in charge of the day gave a lecture using a textbook on chemical biology. After the person lectured on one chapter, all of the other students then discussed the theme.
May, 2011– July, 2011	Community pharmacy practice at Bosei Pharmacy, Kumamoto Activities included: Learning about the duties of a community pharmacy pharmacist. In particular, how to fill a prescription, compounding, drug administration guidance, home medical care, and medical security systems.
September, 2011– December, 2011	Hospital practice at Red Cross Hospital, Kumamoto Activities included: Learning about the duties of a hospital pharmacist: filling prescriptions, dispensing injection drugs, drug administration guidance, and in-patient pharmaceutical service. I also learned about the duties of other health care professionals such as: doctors, nurses, dietitians, radiation technologists, and laboratory technicians.

Work Experience

May, 2008– March, 2012	**UNIGLO, Kumamoto** Duties included: Working as a sales floor staff. I helped support the regular sales staff and then was promoted to sales staff. In 2010, I was able to become an assistant floor manager. I had many responsibilities and learned the importance of being professional at all times.

Computer Skills
MS Word, Excel, Power Point, and Chem Draw

Language Skills
Japanese: Native speaker
English: Scored 930 on the TOEIC (December, 2012)

Licenses
August, 2007　Japanese driver's license

Other
Studied abroad for six weeks in 2011 in America to learn about pharmacy education and practice there.

Kendo (4 dan)−I have been practicing kendo for 15 years and was also the leader of the kendo club of my university in 2009.

Love traveling and meeting other people and am also a member of the International Pharmacy Students' Federation. I attended the conference in 2012 in Egypt.

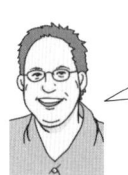

Eric's Tip 13　強気でいこう！

　ネガティブな印象を与えてしまう "I can't...", "I don't like...", "I am unable to..." などを使ってはいけません．代わりに，"I look forward to challenging," や "I have an open mind to new things," あるいは "I will do my best." と表現すれば前向きな印象になります．〔付録 E（p.85）参照〕

II

◆ ◆ ◆ ◆ ◆ ◆ ◆ ◆ ◆

話し方・聞き方

Chapter 8

話し方・聞き方の基本
Speaking／Listening Basics

　これからの社会では，英語で書く能力が重要なのと同じくらいに，英語で話すことも重要になります．しかし，多くの日本人が大切な基本を忘れてしまっているために，不自然な英語を使っています．

　自然な英語を話すために気をつけてほしいことは，**息継ぎ**，**イントネーション**，**話す速さ**の三つです．

8・1　息継ぎ（Your breathing）

　日本語と同じく，英語にも句読点があります．どのタイミングで呼吸すればよいかがわかるので，句読点は重要です．たとえば：

1) ","コンマでは，止めて，半呼吸します．
2) "."ピリオドでは，止めて，一呼吸します．
3) ";"セミコロンでは，止めて，半呼吸と一呼吸の中間くらいの息をします．
4) "?"疑問符では，止めて，一呼吸します．
5) "!"感嘆符では，止めて，一呼吸します．

　一番大切なことですが，コンマやピリオドなどがないところで止めてはいけません．不自然に止めてしまうと，あなたが話している英語をネイティブスピーカーは理解しにくくなってしまいます．

> **Examples**
>
> ① I have been to Boston, New York, and Washington D.C.
> My father, mother, and brother are all pharmacists, too.
> ② I have worked as a tutor. I helped junior high school students learn English.
> His name is Yasuhito. Everyone calls him Yasu.
> ③ The movie was very interesting; it had many surprises.
> The plane was full of people; it was not a good situation.
> ④ Excuse me, can I ask you a question?
> Pardon me, where is the men's room?
> ⑤ Happy birthday to you! Have a great day!
> Merry Xmas! And happy new year!

8・2 イントネーション（抑揚，Intonation）

イントネーションは，発音や文法よりも重要かもしれません．イントネーションを間違えると，誤解につながる可能性が高くなります．

1) "." ピリオドでは，抑揚をつけません［→］．
2) "?" 疑問符では，声を高くします（上昇調）［↗］．
3) "!" 感嘆符では，声を急激に高くします［↗］．

図7を見てみましょう．めがねをかけた男性は友人とレストランに来ています．注文を聞かれ緊張したのか "I would like a hamburger. ↗" と上昇調で答えてしまいました．店員さんは困っていますね．

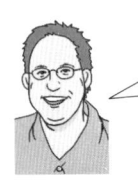

> **Eric's Tip 14　質問時のイントネーション**
>
> 質問をするときは語尾を上げましょう．When, Where, Why, Who, What, Which, Howなどで始まる疑問文は語尾を下げると習ったかもしれませんが，あまり気にすることはありません．ネイティブスピーカーは質問するときに語尾を上げるのが一般的です．

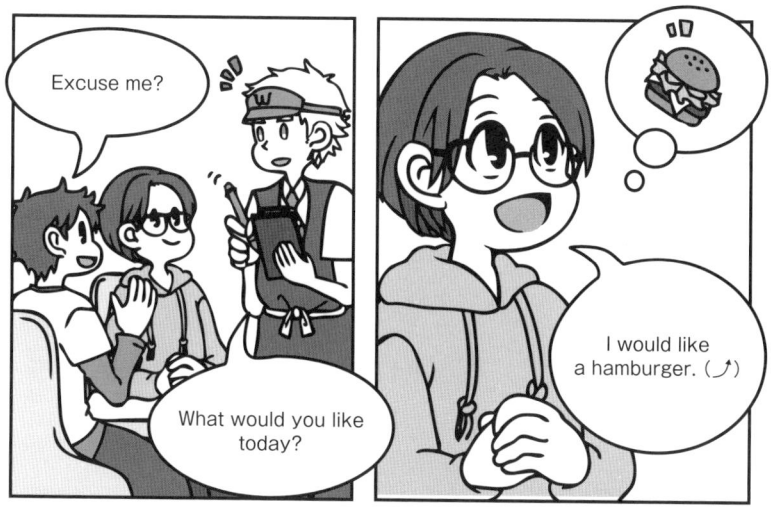

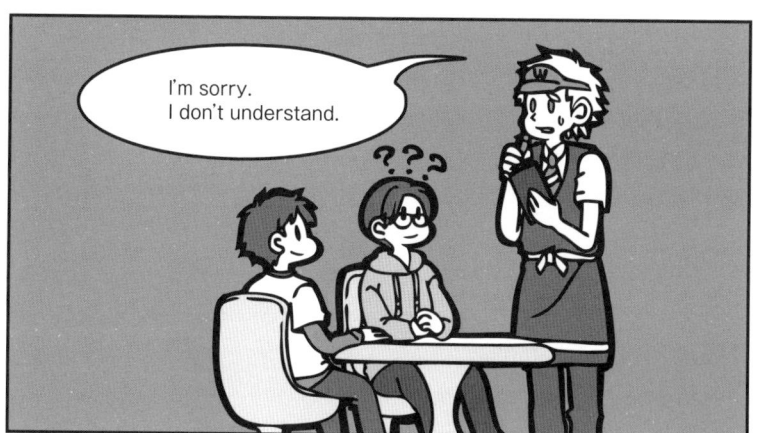

図7　I would like a hamburger（?）

8・3　話す速さ（Speed）

　英語を学習する人の多くが，速く話さなければいけないと思い込んでいるようですが，そんなことはありません．正しい息継ぎとイントネーションで英語を話せば，ゆっくりしゃべっていてもプロらしく聞こえます．

Chapter 9

Please, Thank you, Excuse me の使い方
Please, Thank you, and Excuse me

英語が上手くない人でも，簡単な三つの表現"Please"，"Thank you"，"Excuse me,"を使えば，丁寧にプロらしく話しているように聞こえます．

9・1 "Please"の使い方
誰かに何かをお願いするときは必ず"Please"を使いましょう．たとえば，

Examples 1
① May I use your bathroom, please?
② Please pass the salt and pepper.
③ Please wait a moment.
④ Speak more slowly, please.
⑤ Please repeat that.

Track 4

何かお願いするときには，疑問文のほうが平文よりも丁寧な表現になります．たとえば，"Please pass the salt and pepper."よりも"Could you please pass the salt and pepper?"と言ったほうが丁寧です．また，"Please"は，文の最初に使うこともあれば，最後に使うこともあるので覚えておきましょう．

"Please" の使用パターン

1) Question with please
2) Question without please
3) Sentence with please
4) Sentence
5) One word

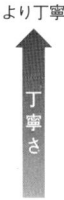

より丁寧 ↑ 丁寧さ

第Ⅰ部でも書きましたが，あなたと相手の人との関係性が重要です．友人に何かお願いするときには，"Please show me your phone." と平文を使います．しかし，相手が自分よりも目上の場合（先生や上司，年上の相手など），平文を使ってはいけません．常に "Could you please show me your phone?" と疑問文を使います．忘れないで下さい．"話し方で人となりがわかる" のです．

9・2 "Thank you" の使い方

誰かに助けてもらったときや，何か物をもらったときには，必ず "thank you" またはより丁寧な "appreciate" と言いましょう．

Examples 2　　　　　　　　　　　　　　　　　　　　　　CD Track 5

① A さん：Sure, the bathroom is over there.
　B さん：Thank you very much.

② A さん：Here you go.
　B さん：Thank you.

③ A さん：OK.
　B さん：Thanks.

④ A さん：I'm sorry. I will speak more slowly from now on.
　B さん：I really appreciate that!

⑤ A さん：Oh. I said that the flight will be delayed one hour due to a storm.
　B さん：I see. Thank you so much.

Useful Expressions

1) I sincerely appreciate that.
2) I really appreciate that.
3) Thank you so much./
   Thank you very much.
4) Thank you.
5) Thanks.

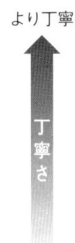

より丁寧 ↑ 丁寧さ

9・3 "Excuse me" の使い方

誰かに何かをお願いするときや助けてもらうときには "Excuse me," を使いましょう． "please" とは違い，常に平文や疑問文の最初に使います．また，"Excuse me," と同じく "pardon me," も自然な英語でよく使います．

Examples 3

CD Track 6

① Excuse me, where is the restroom?
② Excuse me, what time is it?
③ Excuse me, how much does this cost?

"Please" や "Thank you" や "Excuse me," を使うときには，アイコンタクトをとって，大きな声で言いましょう．

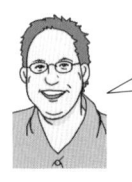

Eric's Tip 15　ドアを通るときのマナー

ドアを開けるときは，すぐ後ろから人が来ていないか確かめましょう．誰か来ていれば，ドアを押さえて先に通ってもらうか，先に通ってドアを押さえておきます．ドアを開けてもらったら，お礼を言って先に通ります．特に日本の男性は，レディーファーストを心がけるようにして下さい．

Chapter 10

挨　拶
"Aisatsu"

　日本語と同様に，英語でも挨拶は重要です．日本語の"おはよう"にあたる"Good morning."は最もよく使う表現です．

　米国のホテルに滞在したとき，筆者の学生たちは知らない人から"Good morning."と挨拶されることに驚いていました．ホームステイであれば，家族に"Good morning."と言うのは常識です．ホテルでも，知らない人同士であっても，挨拶はマナーなのです．

　そのときの時刻に合った挨拶をしましょう．午前10時以降に"Good morning."はちょっと変です．そのころから就寝時間までは，"Hello,"（日本語の"こんにちは"）と言います．英語の"こんにちは"の言い方にはいろいろあります．

こんにちは	Good afternoon.	より丁寧 ↑ 丁寧さ
	Hello.	
	Hi.	
	Hey.	

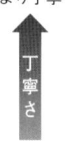

	How's life?	知らない人からこのように聞かれることがあります．本当に何か質問されているわけではないので，立ち止まって丁寧に答える必要はありません．簡単に"OK"と答えておきましょう．
	How are you?	
	What's up?	

　このような言い回しを使うときには，常にアイコンタクトをとって，大きな声で，笑顔で言いましょう．

Examples

① 相手に "Hi, how are you?" と言われた場合

<相手が知らない人なら＞

Fine, thanks.

<相手が友人なら＞

Oh hi, Amanda! Long time, no see! I am OK. I am just so busy. And you? How is Yujiro?

② 相手に "Hi, what's up?" と言われた場合

<相手が知らない人なら＞

Not much.

<相手が友人なら＞

Hi, Kazumi! I was just thinking of you and the new quilt I made. If you are free, please come over to my home and I will show it to you.

③ 相手に "How's life?" と言われた場合

<相手が知らない人なら＞

Pretty good. And you?*

<相手が友人なら＞

Oh, not so good, Michael. I have been a little sick. I had the flu last week and before that I hurt my ankle. How are you?

* 知らない人からの挨拶に対してのみ使う表現です．友人にこのように答えるのは失礼です．

Chapter 11

自然な英語での自己紹介
Introducing Yourself in Natural English

以下は，英語でプロらしく自己紹介をするときに役立つ順番です．

1) 挨　拶（Greeting）： It's a pleasure to meet you.
　　　　　　　　　　　　Nice to meet you.
　　　　　　　　　　　　Hello.
2) 自分の氏名．必要であればスペルも伝えましょう．たとえば，日本語を話さない人に"Ryosuke"は聞き取りにくい名前です．R-Y-O-S-U-K-E とスペルを伝えれば相手は理解しやすくなります．
3) 学生ならば"I am a 5th-year student pharmacist."のような言い方が適切です．"pharmacy student"でも伝わりますが，自然な英語ではありません．

＜ホームステイ先での自己紹介＞

Examples 1

Track 8

① Hello, my name is Atsuko [Shaking hands]. It is spelled A-T-S-U-K-O. I'm a 4th-year student pharmacist. I'm very happy to finally meet you in person. Thank you so much for letting me stay with you.

② Hi, I'm Akihiro. That is spelled A-K-I-H-I-R-O. Please call me Hiro. I will be a 3rd-year student pharmacist from next month. This is my first time to your country and I really appreciate your letting me stay with your lovely family.

<面接試験(就職活動)での自己紹介>

Examples 2

Track 9

① Good afternoon. My name is Yoshito Yamaguchi. I am a 5th-year student pharmacist at Tokyo College of Pharmacy. I am very interested in working in your company in the future. Thank you so much for this opportunity today.

② Good morning. My first name is Yuka and my last name is Shimazaki. I will be a 6th-year student pharmacist from April. I have heard many good things about your company and hope to work for you after I graduate. Thank you for seeing me.

Chapter 12

スモールトーク：
好ましい質問と質問への答え方
Small Talk: Asking Appropriate Questions and Answering Questions

　英国で行われた研究によると，同じ職場で働いている英語のネイティブスピーカーとそうでない人の間で**スモールトーク**がある会社のほうが，業績が上がっているということです．スモールトークはとても重要です．
　スモールトークの第一歩は質問です．とは言っても，好ましい質問をするのは簡単ではありません．たとえば，相手をよく知らないときには，次のような話題は避けましょう．

- お 金（Money）
- 政 治（Politics）
- 年 齢（Age）〔特に女性の場合〕
- 宗 教（Religion）
- 性生活（Sex）

　相手があなたに質問する際にも同じことが言えます．もし初対面の人に"How much did your watch cost?"と聞かれたら，相手はマナーをわきまえていない人だと言えます．あなたから何か盗んでやろうと企んでいるのかもしれません．気をつけて下さい．
　もちろん，友達になろうとしている人であれば，このような話題を取上げても大丈夫です．しかし，時と場合は考えましょう．
　では，どのような話題が適切なのでしょうか．状況にもよりますが，次の1)〜5)は一般的に好ましいとされる話題です．

1) スポーツ (Sports)
2) 家族 (Family)
3) ペット (Pets)
4) 旅行 (Travel)
5) 食べ物 (Food)

12・1　スモールトーク（スポーツ）

日本でもそうであるように，サッカーのようなスポーツは人気があります．スポーツは，相手と仲良くなりたいときにはよい話題です．

Example 1

Aさん：What's your favorite sport?
Bさん：Oh, I like baseball.
Aさん：Which team do you like?
Bさん：I like the New York Yankees. They are very strong.
Aさん：I agree, but I don't like them.
Bさん：Who is your favorite team?
Aさん：I like the L.A.Dodgers.
Bさん：Why do you like them?
Aさん：I am from Los Angeles and I saw many of their games when I was young.
Bさん：I see. That makes sense.

上記は親しい人との丁寧なスモールトークです．丁寧な英語で，好ましい質問で，はじめに質問した人も同じ質問を相手から返されて答えています．

Useful Expressions

1) Who's your favorite baseball/football/soccer team?
2) Do you like to play any sports?
3) What sports do you like to watch?

12・2 スモールトーク（家族）

どこの国の人も，家族の写真をオフィスに置いたり，財布に入れたり，家の壁に飾ったりします．家族の写真を見たら，写真に写っているのは誰か尋ねるのが一般的です．

Example 2　　　　　　　　　　　　　　　　　　　　　Track 11

Aさん：Excuse me, are these your children?
Bさん：Yes, they are.
Aさん：What are their names?
Bさん：They are Alex and Andrew.
Aさん：They are so cute.
Bさん：Thank you. So, do you have any children?
Aさん：Yes, I do. I have two girls: Miho and Miyako.
Bさん：Here's a picture of them with my wife.
Aさん：You have a beautiful family.
Bさん：Thank you.

Useful Expressions

1) Excuse me, are these your children?
2) Excuse me, who is this?
3) Excuse me, is this your husband?
4) Excuse me, who is she?

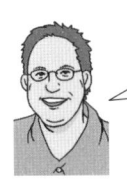

Eric's Tip 16　質問の内容に注意

曖昧・失礼・不必要な質問は避けましょう．"どこから来ましたか？"は曖昧です．"お箸が使えますか？"は失礼です．"納豆はお好きですか？"はどうでもいいことです．

12・3　スモールトーク（ペット）

多くの人がペットを飼っています．愛犬家や愛猫家であれば，ペットの話題を通して友達になれるかもしれません．

Example 3

Aさん：Do you have any pets?
Bさん：Yes, I do. I have two cats.
Aさん：What are their names?
Bさん：Their names are Garfield and Felix. How about you?
Aさん：I have a dog.
Bさん：Is it a boy or a girl?
Aさん：A boy. His name is Fido.
Bさん：What kind of dog is he?
Aさん：He is a poodle.
Bさん：I see.

Useful Expressions

1) Do you like dogs? What kind?
2) Do you have any pets?
3) Do you like any animals?

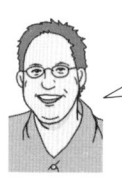

Eric's Tip 17　自分で答えにくい質問は避けましょう

相手の立場に立って質問しましょう．たとえば，恋人について質問したら，同じ質問が自分にも返ってきます．年齢について聞くと，自分の年齢も聞かれます．自分だけ答えないのは非常に失礼です．

12・4　スモールトーク（旅行）

　国際的な企業であれば，社員は旅行好きかもしれません．世界各国への旅行についての話題は，会話のきっかけになるはずです．

Example 4

Track 13

Aさん：Is this your first time to America?
Bさん：No, it isn't. It is my third time.
Aさん：Where else have you visited?
Bさん：I have been to New York and Washington D.C.
Aさん：Have you been to any other countries?
Bさん：Many. I have been to Europe, the Middle East, and Africa, too. And you?
Aさん：I haven't traveled so much. I want to go to Europe though.
Bさん：You should! France, Italy, Switzerland...they are all beautiful countries!
Aさん：Sounds great! I hope to go soon.

Useful Expressions

1) Do you like to travel? Which countries have you been to?
2) Which part of America/Europe/Asia do you recommend I visit?
3) Where do you recommend I stay?

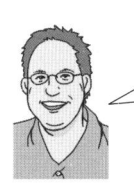

Eric's Tip 18　"hate" は使ってはダメ！

　嫌いな食べ物について話すとき，"I hate 〜" という表現は，相手に悪い印象を与えます．"I am sorry, but I do not like 〜." のほうが，丁寧な印象になります．

12・5　スモールトーク（食べ物）

旅行と同じく，さまざまな国の食べ物に関する話題は，よいスモールトークになります．東京のような多くの首都には，世界中のおいしい食べ物があります．タイ，中国，インド，日本，フランス，米国の料理などは，適切なスモールトークの話題です．

Example 5

Track 14

Aさん：Would you like to get something to eat?
Bさん：Sure! What do you recommend?
Aさん：Do you have a food preference?
Bさん：I eat anything. And you?
Aさん：I eat all kinds of food, too. How about Indian food?
Bさん：Oh, I love curry!
Aさん：Great! I know a nice little shop near here.
Bさん：OK. Let's go.

Useful Expressions

1) Do you have a food preference?
2) Do you have any food allergies? *
3) Do you like to cook?

＊　誰かを食事に招待したり，一緒に外食に出かけたりする前に，このように質問して確かめておきましょう．

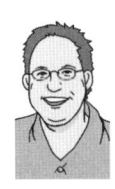

Eric's Tip 19
知っておきたい
海外生活のマナーと表現

◪ホームステイ先で
●ホストファミリーへのお礼

　ホストファミリーの多くはボランティアです．ホームステイ中は常に行儀よく振る舞うように心がけましょう．お世話になるお礼として，日本から何か持参することをお勧めします．決して高価なプレゼントを準備する必要はありません．気の利いた日本的なお土産で十分に感謝の気持ちは伝わります．料理が得意ならば，日本食（天ぷら／焼き鳥／手巻き寿司など）を作って食べていただいても良いですね．

●ホームステイ先ではまず聞いてみよう

　ホームステイ先で何かを借りたり使ったりするのは，ホストファミリーの許可を必ず得てからにしましょう．許可を得る際は"Excuse me,"で始めます．たとえば次のように言います．

Excuse me, may I use the bathroom? （トイレをお借りしてよろしいですか．）
　　　　　 may I wash my clothes? （服を洗濯させていただけますか．）
　　　　　 may I get something to drink? （飲み物をいただいてもいいですか．）

　わからないことや困ったことは，躊躇せずに聞いてみましょう．

●ホストファミリーへのお礼状

　ホームステイの最終日，ホストファミリーにお礼状を渡すことをお勧めします．素敵な和紙のカードを日本から持参する，あるいは滞在先で事前に購入して準備しておきましょう．カードには"Thank you."で感謝の気持ちを記すほか，どんなことが嬉しかったのかを具体的に書きましょう．一例を示すと，

　Thank you so much for everything while I stayed with you.
　　In particular, I sincerely enjoyed our talks about life.
　　　　　　　（人生についてお話できて楽しかった．）
　　　　　　　I really loved the meals you cooked for me.
　　　　　　　（手料理がとてもおいしかった．）
　　　　　　　it was wonderful spending time with your beautiful family.
　　　　　　　（素敵なご家族と一緒に時間を過ごせて良かった．）

🔲 チップのマナー
● チップはいる？ いらない？
　チップに関してややこしく感じることがあるかもしれません．たとえば，サーバー（ウェイターやウェイトレスは古い英語のため今は使われません）のいないカフェやコーヒーショップでのチップは不要ですが，レジの近くにチップ入れを置いてある店があります．チップ入れに気づいたら，あまっている小銭やおつりを入れるようにしましょう．とはいっても，気持ちの良いサービスを受けたと思えるときだけです．サーバーがいなくてチップ入れも見当たらなければ，チップは不要です．

● 良いサービスには多めのチップ
　米国のレストランで良いサービスをしてもらったら，チップを渡すのは当然です．非常に良いサービスならば 20%，まあまあ良いサービスならば 10〜15%．サービスが悪ければチップは不要です．

● 道順を教えてもらったらチップ
　海外での旅行中は，見知らぬ人に道を尋ねたり何かお願いをしたりしないほうが無難です．その代わり食事で利用するレストランのサーバーに聞いてみましょう．サーバーが親切に対応してくれたら，チップを少し上乗せして渡します．たとえば，道に迷って，探している場所が見つからないときに，サーバーが道順を教えてくれたら，チップは少し多めに払います．

🔲 レストランでのマナー
● 十人十色で OK
　日本では何人もの人が同じ料理を注文します．しかしこれは，他の国の人にはとても奇妙に映ります．他の人の注文は気にしないで，自分が好きな料理を注文しましょう．

● 注文に悩んだらおススメを聞いてみる
　何を注文したらよいかわからないときは，サーバーに"本日のおススメ (Today's special)"を聞いてみましょう．おススメが本当においしかったら，チップを少し多めに渡しましょう．

● 食事のペースを考える
　自分の注文した料理が先に来たら，他の人の分が揃うまで待っている必要はありません．だからと言って，あまり急いで食べてしまうのもダメです．少しだけ食べておいて，他の人と一緒に食べ終わるようにしましょう．

Eric's Tip 19 知っておきたい海外生活のマナーと表現

●手で食べても OK

多くの米国料理は"フィンガーフード"とよばれているように，直接手で持って食べて OK です．フライドポテト，ハンバーガー，サンドイッチ，スペアリブ，タコスなどは典型的なフィンガーフードです．

◧買い物のマナー：店員さんとの会話

買い物に行き，店員さんと話をする際は，まずアイコンタクトをとってからにしましょう．レジでは，"Is this everything for today ?" や "Did you find everything you were looking for ?" などの質問に答える心づもりが必要です．といっても，これらは文字どおりの質問ではなく，接客に使われる挨拶の一種です．いずれにせよ，客側は何か言わなくてはいけませんから，"Yes, it is." や "Yes, I did, thank you." と答えます．もちろん，探していたものが見つからなかった場合は，助けを求める絶好の機会です．"Actually, where is your 〜 ?" や "Do you sell 〜 ?" と聞いてみましょう．

◧日常生活のマナー
●身分証明書（ID）携帯は常識

クレジットカードを使って支払いをするとき，アルコールを購入するとき，ホテルへのチェックイン時など，海外での旅行中は "Please show me some ID." と ID（身分証明書）の提示をたびたび求められます．観光目的での滞在中のおもな ID はパスポートです．ですから，常にパスポートを携帯する必要があります．ズボンの後ろポケットに無造作に入れておくなんて危険です．落としたりスラれたりしないように，とにかく気をつけましょう．

●国際学生証はお得

いろんな国に学生割引の制度があります．海外で学生割引を利用するには，大学生であることを示す ID が必要ですが，日本語の学生証では通用しません．そこで海外旅行の出発前に，世界共通の学生身分証明書である国際学生証（International Student Identity Card）を取得しておきましょう（詳しくは http://www.isic.jp/）．この ID を提示することで，ホテルの宿泊代，運賃，美術館や博物館の入場料，遊園地の入場料などがかなり節約できます．

●携帯電話のマナー

日本と違って，公けの場所での携帯電話の使用やマナーに関して，海外ではあまりうるさく言わないようです．だからと言って，レストランでの食事中，学校で授業を受けている最中および，誰かとの会話中や，静かな雰囲気の場所では，

よほどの緊急時でない限り，携帯電話は使わないようにしましょう．他の人たちと一緒にいるときに携帯電話を使うならば，他の人から離れて戸外に出たり，トイレや静かな場所に移動したりしましょう．このとき "Excuse me," と言って席を立ちましょう．

● Wi-Fi（無線 LAN）は使える？
驚くかもしれませんが，Wi-Fi（無線 LAN）は海外では有料かそんなに簡単にはアクセスできません．コーヒーショップや大学構内など限られた場所の Wi-Fi が無料で使える国は増えてきました．しかし，ホテルの Wi-Fi 使用は有料になることが多いので気をつけましょう．宿泊する前にホテルのポリシーを確認しておくとよいでしょう．Wi-Fi が無料かどうかを話題にするとき，"free" とは言いません．一般的に使われる単語は "complimentary" です．

◆知っておきたい単語の使い分け
● "learn" と "study"
英語の "learn" には熟達や精通といったニュアンスがあります．たとえば，"I learned how to ride a bike." は，自転車の乗り方を習得していることを意味します．ですから "I learned English for six years." と言うと，英語を6年間で習得した，つまり話せるという意味になりますが，実際にはどうでしょうか．学習したものの熟達しているわけではないときは "study" を使い，"I studied English for six years." と言います．自分自身のことを書いたり，これまでに自分は何を学んできたのかを書いたりするとき，特に気をつけましょう．

● "practice" と "play"
楽器や武道を話題にするとき，英語では "play" よりも "practice" を使います．たとえば，"I play the violin in my free time." よりも "I like to practice the violin in my free time." のほうがベターな表現になります．"play the violin" というと，プロの音楽家のように聞こえるからです．たいていは "practice" のほうが無難です．空手，柔道，剣道，合気道といった武道もすべて，"play" ではなく "practice" です．

● 自分の研究について話すとき
"I research ～." は，間違いではありませんが，正確な英語ではありません．実験室で行っている自分の研究について話す際は，"I conduct research on ～." のように言いましょう．もっと良い表現は，"I investigate ～." です．このような表現を使えば，文法的に正しく，プロらしい英語に聞こえます．

Chapter 13

ネイティブスピーカーの英語の発音
Native Speaker's Pronunciation

13・1 言葉 (Words)

日本人はあまり知らないのですが，最も典型的なネイティブスピーカーの英語の発音には以下の 1 ～ 3 があります．

1 t が二つ重なれば，大抵の場合 d のように発音します．
　・"better" は "*beder*" と発音します．
　・"letter" は "*leder*" と発音します．

> **Examples 1**　　　　　　　　　　　　　　　　　　　　　Track 15
> ① I think this one is better than that one.
> ② I will send you the letter today. You will get it in two days.

2 t が一つでも，単語の真ん中にある場合は，d のように発音します．
　・"water" は自然な英語では "*wader*" と発音します．

> **Example 2**　　　　　　　　　　　　　　　　　　　　　Track 16
> Excuse me, can I have a glass of water?

3 以下は（米国人の場合の）母音の自然な発音です．短い単語では，前置詞や代名詞の発音が変わります．

　・"to" は "ta"，"you" は "ya" と発音します．

> **Examples 3**　　　　　　　　　　　　　　　　　　　　CD Track 17
> ① I would like to have a non-smoking room, please.
> ② Can you pass the salt and pepper?

アメリカ英語では，母音の a, e, i, o, u, はすべて "a" の発音になります．英国とオーストラリアでは母音の発音は異なります．とにかく米国人は "a" が大好きです．

> **Examples 4**　　　　　　　　　　　　　　　　　　　　CD Track 18
> ① This is my brother. His name is Alex and he lives in Boston.
> ② Anything from Korea is quite popular in Japan now.

13・2　二つ以上の言葉（Sets of Words）

自然な英語では，二つや三つの単語を一緒に発音するので，聞き取るのが非常に難しいかもしれません．"Nicetameecha（Nice to meet you）" はその一例です．

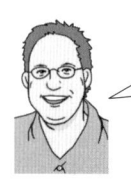

> **Eric's Tip 20　初心者は使わないほうがイイ**
> ネイティブスピーカーのまねをして "beder"，"leder" と発音すると，ネイティブスピーカーはあなたは英語が上手だと判断して速く話してしまうかもしれません．初心者のうちは "better" や "letter" と発音しておきましょう．

Chapter 13 ネイティブスピーカーの英語の発音

Examples 5　　　　　　　　　　　　　　　　　　　　　CD Track 19

① Would you＝woudja　　⑥ Want to＝wanna
② Did you＝didja　　　　⑦ Going to＝gonna
③ Could you＝couldja　　⑧ Aren't you＝arencha
④ Can't you＝cantcha　　⑨ Nice to meet you＝nicetameecha
⑤ Have to＝hafta

　　　③ Could you please say that again?
　　　⑥ I want to see you on the 19th of next month.
　　　⑦ We are going to reevaluate the project.

自然な英語で一番注意しておきたいのは，h の発音です．基本的に h は発音しません．h で始まる代名詞（he, his, him, her, hers）が文の途中にあるときには，その前の単語とくっつけて発音します．

[1]　"I **think his** name is Eric." は "I **thinkis** name is Eric." と発音します．"his" の "h" は発音せずに，残りの "is" はその前の "think" とくっつけて発音します．

[2]　"Will you **ask her** a question for me?" は "Will you **asker** a question for me?" と発音します．

[3]　"I **called him** yesterday." は "I **calledim** yesterday." と発音します．

Examples 6　　　　　　　　　　　　　　　　　　　　　CD Track 20

① I think his name is Eric.
② Will you ask her a question for me?
③ I called him yesterday.
④ I will go to the conference with him.
⑤ I talked with her about the problem.
⑥ He said it wasn't his umbrella.

自然な英語では，"and" や "but" の接続詞は，前後の単語にくっつけて発音します．たとえば，

4 "I would like some **salt and pepper**, please." は "I would like some **salt'npepper**, please." と発音します．

5 "I have **been to** America many times, **but I** still can't understand English well." は "I have **beenta** America many times, **budi** still can't understand English well." と発音します．

> **Examples 7**　　　　　　　　　　　　　CD Track 21
> ① I would like some salt and pepper, please.
> ② I have been to America many times, but I still can't understand English well.
> ③ It was raining cats and dogs, means it was raining very hard.
> ④ My friend is a good worker, but he drinks too much.

13・3　短縮形（Contractions）

短縮形も自然な英語でよく使われます．英語を書くときには，

"cannot"　　"do not"　　"they are"

と綴るのが普通です．しかし，英語を話すときには，

"can't"　　"don't"　　"they're"

と短縮します．英語を話すときにはたいてい，短縮形を使います．

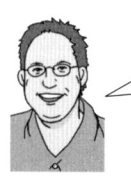

> **Eric's Tip 21　聞き取れないときは丁寧に聞き返す**
> ネイティブスピーカーの発音が聞き取れないとき「エッ？」と日本語で返事をするのは止めましょう．"Excuse me,"とか"Pardon me,"または"I am sorry, could you repeat that?"と丁寧に言って，もう一度話してもらいましょう．

Examples 8

<短縮形>

	短縮形		短縮形
Cannot	Can't	It would	It'd
Did not	Didn't	That would	That'd
Could not	Couldn't	They would	They'd
Was not	Wasn't	He would	He'd
Will not	Won't	She would	She'd
They are	They're	I will	I'll
You are	You're	You will	You'll
How are	How're	That will	That'll
What are	What're	They will	They'll
Where are	Where're	It will	It'll
I am	I'm		
He is	He's		
She is	She's		
That is	That's		
There is	There's		

Chapter 14

面　接
Interviews

　面接では誰もが緊張しがちです．しかし，自分のことを相手によく知ってもらえる絶好の機会です．アイコンタクトをしっかりととって，丁寧な言葉で，はっきりと正直に質問に答えましょう．けっしてネガティブなことを言ってはいけません．自分の将来の可能性をアピールしましょう．

＜面接の例 1＞

Track 23

面接者： Hello, my name is Michael Ramsey and I am vice president of personnel of the Swiss Pharmaceutical Corporation. I am here to interview you today. Ready?

志望者： Yes, sir.

面接者： First, please share a little about yourself.

志望者： Well, my name is Sachiko Tanaka, please call me Sachiko. I have an older brother and a younger sister. I belong to the clinical pharmacy lab and I am interested in doing research on new therapies for organ transplants. When I have free time, I play the violin and was the concert mistress of my university's orchestra.

面接者： Very impressive! I also love classical music, but can't play any instruments. By the way, what interests you in our company?

志望者： I am interested in working for your company as it is doing cutting-edge research that I hope to be involved with in the

Chapter 14 面　　接　　　　　　　67

面接者： future. I think that working for your company could allow me to grow and help make new drugs to help many people.

面接者： That is very kind of you, Sachiko. Lastly, would you be able to relocate to one of our research centers in America, Switzerland, or India?

志望者： I think so. I have never lived abroad, but I have traveled and have done two homestays: one in New Zealand and another in Boston. I love meeting new people and learning about new cultures.

面接者： Excellent! Well, thank you for coming to the interview today, Sachiko. We are still going to interview some others, but we should be in touch with you in the coming days.

志望者： Thank you, Mr. Ramsey. I look forward to hearing from you.

＜面接の例 2＞

Track 24

面接者： Good afternoon, my name is Colleen Spates and I am senior vice president for personnel for the British Pharmaceutical Corporation. I am here to ask you a few questions. Are you ready?

志望者： Yes, I am.

面接者： First, tell me a little about yourself.

志望者： My name is Kohei Ito, please call me Kohei. I am the youngest child and have two sisters. I have played baseball since I was 6 and was the captain of the baseball team at my university. My favorite subject is organic chemistry and I also like English. When I have free time, I like to travel and have been to more than 20 different countries.

面接者：	I see. Twenty countries?! That's very impressive. Which country was your favorite to visit?
志望者：	Last summer I drove with my friends more than 6,000 kilometers across America－that was a great experience!
面接者：	Sounds like you had quite the experience! And what appeals to you about our company?
志望者：	When I learned more about your company, I liked how there are opportunities for advancement and travel. I think your future product line is going to be a very good one, too.
面接者：	What a nice thing to say. Speaking of travel, what are your thoughts about relocating abroad?
志望者：	Actually, I would be more than happy to relocate. I am fine working in Japan, but I am also comfortable living abroad. I grew up in Singapore and Thailand and think I would be able to live in many different countries.
面接者：	I see. Thank you, Kohei, for your time today. We will be in touch in the coming days.
志望者：	And thank you, Ms. Spates! I look forward to hearing from you.

III

プレゼンテーションの上達法
Better Presentation Skills

Chapter 15

プレゼンテーションの上達法
Better Presentation Skills

　製薬会社に就職しても，研究者になっても，病院や薬局の薬剤師になっても，誰でも一度はプレゼンテーションを経験するはずです．

　プレゼンテーションが上手だと，明るい将来が約束されるかもしれません．逆にプレゼンテーションが下手だと，かなり苦労することになるかもしれません．英語圏では，プロらしいプレゼンテーションをする能力がとても重視されています．

　プレゼンテーションの際に，覚えておきたいことを以下に示します．

1. 緊張しないようにすること．誰でも緊張しますが，リラックスするように心がけることが重要です．どうすれば緊張しなくなるのでしょうか．練習あるのみです．プレゼンテーションを何度もするうちに，緊張しなくなります．

2. 人に話をするときのように，大きな声で，可能な限りアイコンタクトをとること．思い出して下さい．英語のコミュニケーションでは，伝える責任は話し手にあります．聞き手ではないのです．

3. プレゼンテーションを準備するときには，まず聞き手のことを考慮すること．聞き手は誰なのか．自分と同じ年齢層か．教育背景はどうか．性別は？といったことが重要になります．これらを考えてみることで，どのような英語を使えばよいかがわかります．英語が堪能な聞き手であれば，専門的な英語を使っても大丈夫です．英語をあまり得意としない聞き手のときには，わかりやすい英語を使いましょう．

4 構成は，はじめの挨拶，内容，結びの挨拶，の三部構成で行うこと．挨拶で始めて，最後にも挨拶を忘れないようにしましょう．

5 パワーポイントを使うときには，1枚の画面にあまり多くの文章を書かないこと．シンプルな画像でも効果的なプレゼンテーションになります．

6 スライドの文章を読まないこと．プロらしいプレゼンテーションでは，決して読んではいけません．

7 1枚目のスライドにはプレゼンテーションのタイトル，発表者の氏名，所属を必ず入れること．

8 その次のスライドには，自分と聞き手にプレゼンテーションの内容がわかるように，概要を入れること．概要には少なくとも次のような項目を入れます．

 1 はじめに（Introduction）

 2 内容1（Content 1）
    内容2（Content 2）
    内容3（Content 3）
      ⋮

 3 結 論（Conclusion）

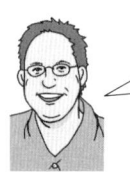

Eric's Tip 22　立ち振る舞いにも気をつけましょう
　マナーに気をつけましょう．大切なプレゼンや面接の最中は，不必要に体には触れないようにしましょう（体を掻く，髪を触る，鼻をこするなど）．公けの場所で必要以上に髪を触ったり，化粧したりするのも止めましょう．

科学的/学際的なプレゼンテーションの概要には以下の項目が含まれます．

1) はじめに/背景（Introduction/Background）
2) 方 法（Materials and methods）
3) 結 果（Results）
4) 考 察（Discussion）
5) 結 論（Conclusion）

9 謝辞．プレゼンテーションの最後に，研究やプレゼンテーションを手助けしてくれた人々に感謝の気持ちを伝えること．"Thank you."と言うのを忘れないようにしましょう．これは最低限のマナーです．

10 最後は結びの挨拶で終えること．英語は"Thank you for your time."です．"Thank you for listening."は自然な英語ではありません．

Useful Expressions

1) はじめの挨拶（Greeting）

> Good morning,
> Good afternoon,
> Good evening,

> First, I appreciate your attending my presentation.
> First, thank you so much for attending.
> First, thanks for coming today.

2) 本 文

> In this slide, we can see ...
> ("On this slide,"ではなく"In this slide,"が正しい英語表現です．)
> Lastly, I wish to thank ... for his/her/their help with the ...
> Lastly, I would like to thank ... for his/her/their help with the ...

3) 結びの挨拶（Final greeting）

> Thank you for your time.

▶ **Checklist** ☑

- ☐ プレゼンテーションの三部構成に沿っているか．
  (Have you followed the fish format for your presentation?)
- ☐ 専門的なパワーポイントか（文字よりも写真/図/表が多いか）．
  〔Are your slides professional? (less text and more pictures/graphs/charts)〕
- ☐ プレゼンテーションに使うパソコンを事前にチェックしたか．
  (Have you checked the computer you will use for your presentation?)
- ☐ 自分のパソコンを持参する必要があるか．
  (Will you need to bring your own?)
- ☐ プレゼンテーションは他のパソコンでも問題なく動作するか．
  (Will your slides work on a different computer?)
- ☐ 自分のパソコンを使用する場合，接続用のアダプターが必要かどうか．
  (If you bring your own computer, make sure whether or not you need an adapter or not?)
- ☐ 表題のパワーポイントを準備したか．
  (Have you prepared a good title slide?)
- ☐ 概要のパワーポイントを準備したか．
  (Have you prepared an outline slide?)
- ☐ 手伝ってくれた人々への謝辞を含めたか．
  (Do you say thank you to the people who helped you?)

次は，プレゼンテーションの一例です．

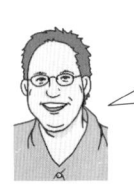

Eric's Tip 23　くしゃみ，咳，あくび

くしゃみをするときには，口を手（できればハンカチ）で覆いましょう．咳が出ているときにも同じです．咳が止まらないときは，退室するのが常識です．あくびをするときも手で口を覆いましょう．食事中の会話でも，口の中に食べ物を入れたまま話すのは止めましょう．

The Issue of Drug Lag in Japan

Track 26

Good morning everyone. Thank you for your time today. I am very happy to share with you about my experience in the U.S. where I visited a school of pharmacy and then learned about an important issue for Japan: drug lag.（スライド1）

スライド1

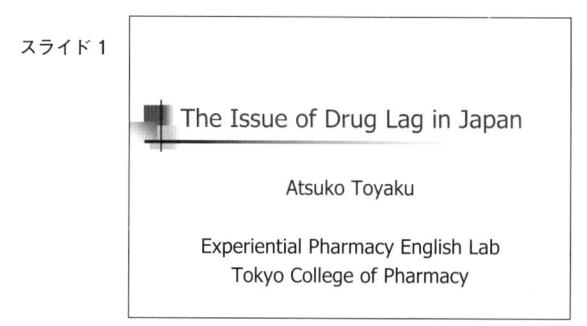

> **The Issue of Drug Lag in Japan**
>
> Atsuko Toyaku
>
> Experiential Pharmacy English Lab
> Tokyo College of Pharmacy

First, I will share about my visit to a school of pharmacy in Los Angeles and the differences in pharmacy practice and education between America and Japan. After that I will talk about drug lag. I will explain what it is and propose some ways for it to be dealt with in Japan.（スライド2）

スライド2

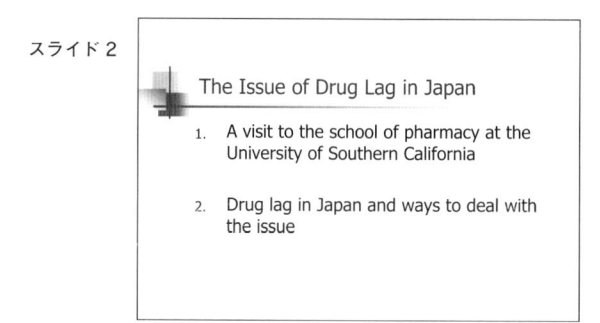

> **The Issue of Drug Lag in Japan**
>
> 1. A visit to the school of pharmacy at the University of Southern California
> 2. Drug lag in Japan and ways to deal with the issue

When I visited the school of pharmacy, I was able to learn about the curriculum for pharmacy schools in California from some professors. I was also able to learn about student life from actual students. It was quite interesting.

This is a picture of a pharmacy on the campus of the university I visited. They sold many OTC drugs and even had a consultation center. In the next slide, here is a sign that says I can get a flu shot in the pharmacy. In America, pharmacists are allowed to give flu shots to patients. This helps keep costs down and means that people don't have to go to a hospital for a flu shot. It is a win-win for many people. (スライド3, スライド4)

スライド3

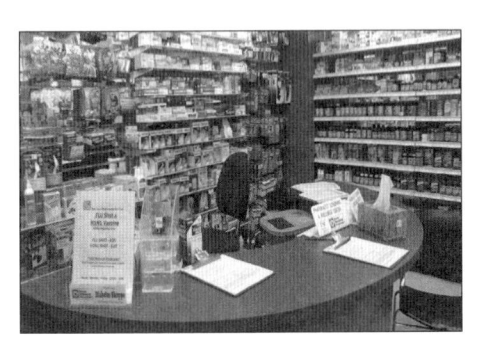

スライド4

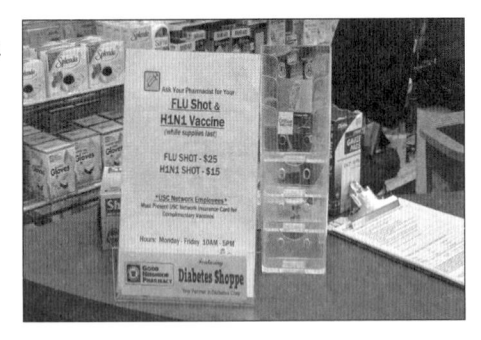

Next, I was able to visit a pharmaceutical company in southern California. It was very interesting. There I met many employees in different fields: drug development, regulatory affairs, and sales. One man, Mr. Yoshida, was very helpful and told me about the differences in getting a new drug to market in America and one in Japan. The time in America was much shorter than in Japan and his company was very happy with the FDA. Since the time to get approved in Japan is much longer, this is called "drug lag". The difference in cost was also very big. As such, it is much easier to do clinical trials in other countries than it is in Japan.（スライド5）

スライド5

> **The Issue of Drug Lag**
> - What is Drug Lag?
> - Why is it happening in Japan?
> 1. Lack of infrastructure and personnel with English skills for timely approval
> 2. Cost of a clinical trial in Japan is too high!

To help overcome the issue of drug lag, I think the following has to be done:（スライド6）

スライド6

> **Ways to Deal with Drug Lag**
> 1. Global cooperation on clinical trials with hospitals and drug companies abroad
> 2. Compassionate use law
> 3. Fast track approval process for new drugs

1. We need to do more clinical trials with companies and hospitals in other countries. To make that possible, though, we need better English education. Right now few Japanese have the ability to use English professionally in clinical trial settings.

2. Second, I think we need a "Compassionate Use" law like they have in America and in European countries to give patients who are critically ill the chance to receive medicines—even if they are not allowed for general use. With their permission, it would allow them to possibly get better sooner and give us data we need to help decide if the medicine would be safe for the people of Japan.

3. Lastly, I hope we can get a "fast track" approval process for medicines for diseases such as AIDS where the patient may not have

long to live. If medicines have been shown to be safe in other countries' studies, this "fast track" approval process would help those medicines enter the market here much faster than the current situation.

In the end, I learned a lot in my 10-day visit to America. I saw what pharmacy education is like, visited a drug company, and learned about the issue of drug lag. In all, I had a wonderful learning experience and wish to thank my professor for having taken me there.（スライド7）

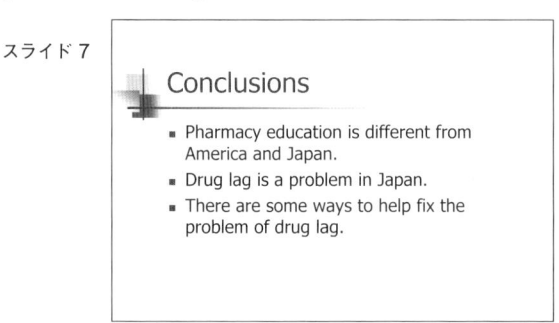

スライド7

Conclusions

- Pharmacy education is different from America and Japan.
- Drug lag is a problem in Japan.
- There are some ways to help fix the problem of drug lag.

I also wish to thank you for attending my presentation today. Any questions?

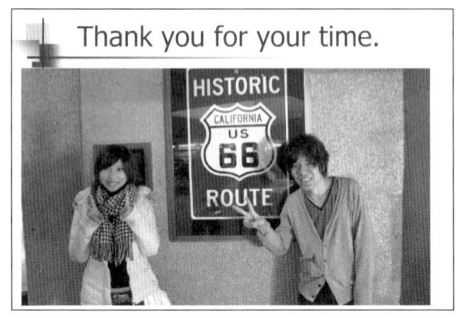

Thank you for your time.（スライド8）

スライド8

Thank you for your time.

付　　録

付録A：薬学領域の科目名
付録B：薬学に関する職業
付録C：薬局・病院でよく使われる
　　　　単語，頭字語，略語
付録D：薬局・病院でよく使われる
　　　　ラテン語由来の略語
付録E：短所を長所に変える表現
　　　　（履歴書向け）

付録 A　薬学領域の科目名

英　語	日　本　語	英　語	日　本　語
Analytical Chemistry	分析化学	Natural Products Chemistry	天然物化学
Anatomy	解剖学	Neuroscience	神経科学
Biochemistry	生化学	Organic Chemistry	有機化学
Bioinformatics	バイオインフォマティクス	Pathology	病理学
Biology	生物学	Pharmaceutics	製剤学
Cell Biology	細胞生物学	Pharmacokinetics	薬物動態学
Chemistry	化　学	Pharmacology	薬理学
Drug Information	医薬品情報学	Pharmacotherapeutics	薬物治療学
Embryology	発生学	Physical Chemistry	物理化学
English	英　語	Physics	物理学
Environmental Science	環境科学	Physiology	生理学
Genetics	遺伝学	Public Health	公衆衛生学
Immunology	免疫学	Radiology	放射線科学
Inorganic Chemistry	無機化学	Regulatory Science	レギュラトリーサイエンス
Math	数　学	Science	科　学
Microbiology	微生物学	Statistics	統計学
Molecular Biology	分子生物学		

付録 B　薬学に関する職業

① hospital pharmacist ［病院薬剤師］
② drugstore pharmacist ［薬局薬剤師（ドラッグストア）］
③ work in a community pharmacy ［薬局薬剤師（調剤薬局）］
④ a pharmacist specializing in ＿＿＿＿＿［＿＿＿＿専門薬剤師］
　（＿＿＿＿には sports, diabetes, chinese herbal medicine, cancer などが入る）
⑤ work as a medical representative（MR）［医薬情報担当者］
⑥ work as a drug representative（DR）［医薬品販売員］
⑦ work in a large pharmaceutical company ［大手製薬会社］
⑧ work in an international drug company ［国際製薬会社］
⑨ work in drug development ［(企業での) 新薬開発・創薬研究］
⑩ work in a contract research organization（CRO）［臨床開発業務受託機関］
⑪ work as a clinical research associate（CRA）［臨床開発モニター］
⑫ work in regulatory affairs ［規制関連業務］
⑬ work in research ［研究者］
⑭ work in education ［大学の先生］

● "～の職に就きたい" という場合は，以下のように下線部に ①～⑭ を入れて表現する．

　①, ②, ④ の場合：I want to be a ＿＿＿＿＿＿＿
　（例）① I want to be a hospital pharmacist.
　　　　④ I want to be a pharmacist specializing in cancer.

　③, ⑤～⑭ の場合：I want to ＿＿＿＿＿＿＿
　（例）⑤ I want to work as a medical representative（MR）.
　　　　⑧ I want to work in an international drug company.

付録 C　薬局・病院でよく使われる単語，頭字語，略語[†]

＜米国に行く前に覚えておきたいおもな単語，頭字語，略語＞

●単　　語
- Medicare　メディケア，高齢者向け医療保険制度
- Medicaid　メディケイド，低所得者向け医療費補助制度
- Medication, drug, medicine, meds　薬剤

●頭 字 語
- BP　　　blood pressure　血圧
- DM　　　diabetes mellitus　糖尿病
- EMT　　emergency medical technician　救命救急士
- FH　　　family history　家族歴
- HTN　　hypertension　高血圧
- MD　　　medical doctor　医師
  〔MD は doctor of medicine 医学(博)士を意味することもある〕
- NKDA　no known drug allergies　薬物アレルギーの既往なし
- OTC　　over-the-counter　処方せんなしで購入できる，店頭販売の，市販の
- P　　　　pulse　脈拍（脈拍数 pulse rate を PR と略すこともある）
- PMH　　prior/previous medical history　既往歴
- RN　　　registered nurse　看護師，(登録)正看護師，公認看護師
- SH　　　social history　社会歴
- T　　　　temperature　体温
- Wt　　　weight　体重

[†]　使用してもよい頭字語や略語を決めている病院や医療機関もあるので，カルテなどに記載する際には，それぞれの機関の指示に従うようにしましょう．

付録 D 薬局・病院でよく使われるラテン語由来の略語[†]

- AC   "ante cibum" ＝ before meals   食前
- PC   "post cibum" ＝ after meals   食後
- Ad lib   "ad libitum" ＝ use as much as one desires; freely   適宜
- BID   "bis in die" ＝ twice a day, two times a day   1 日 2 回
- TID   "ter in die" ＝ three times a day   1 日 3 回
- PO   "per os" ＝ per oral   経口
- HS   "hora somni" ＝ at bedtime   就寝前
- Q   "quaque" ＝ every   ～ごと
- QD   "quaque die" ＝ every day   毎日
  （ただし，QOD や qds と間違えやすいので，安全のために"every day"や"daily"と表現する場所が増えてきている）
- QH   "quaque hora" ＝ every hour   毎時間
- Q 4 hr.   "quaque 4 hora" ＝ every 4 hours   4 時間ごと
- QID   "quater in die" ＝ four times daily   1 日 4 回
- QOD   "quaque one die" ＝ every other day   1 日おきに，隔日
- Rx   "recipe" に由来．処方薬，処方薬のシンボル

[†] 使用してもよい略語を決めている病院や医療機関もあるので，カルテなどに記載する際には，それぞれの機関の指示に従うようにしましょう．

付録 E　短所を長所に変える表現（履歴書向け）

Weakness	短　　所	Strength	長　　所
I am shy.	私は引っ込み思案だ	I am quiet and a deep thinker.	私は静かで物事を深く考える
I don't know how to ~	私は〜のやり方を知らない	I am a quick learner.	私は物覚えがいい
I am not a leader.	私はリーダーではない	I am a team player.	私はチームプレーヤーだ
I am conservative.	私は保守的だ	I am traditionally minded.	私は伝統を重んじる
I don't have much work experience.	私には実務経験があまりない	I am fresh and open to new challenges.	私はフレッシュで新たな挑戦を歓迎する
People think I am strange.	人は私を変わり者だと言う	I am a free-thinker and don't mind being different from others.	私は自由な考えをもち、他の人と違うことを気にしない
I am stubborn.	私は頑固だ	Once I make a decision, I stick to it.	私はいったん決めたことは貫き通す
I am indecisive.	私は優柔不断だ	I like to hear many opinions before making a decision.	私は何か決断する前に、たくさんの意見を聞きたい
I have never left Japan.	私は日本から出たことがない	I look forward to traveling around the world in the future.	私はこれから世界中を旅するのを楽しみにしている
My grades were not so good.	私は成績があまり良くなかった	In college, I was very active with my studies, part-time job, and club activities.	私は在学中、勉学とアルバイトとクラブ活動に積極的に取組んだ
I am an only child.	私は一人っ子だ	I come from a loving family.	私は愛情に満ちた家庭で育った
I am loud and noisy.	私は騒がしい	I am an extrovert and like to communicate with others.	私は外交的で他の人と話をするのが好きだ

第 1 版 第 1 刷 2013 年 6 月 14 日 発 行

薬学生のための実践英語

Ⓒ 2013

著　者　Eric M. Skier
　　　　上　鶴　重　美

発行者　小　澤　美奈子

発　行　株式会社 東京化学同人
東京都文京区千石 3-36-7(〒112-0011)
電話 03-3946-5311・FAX 03-3946-5316
URL: http://www.tkd-pbl.com/

印刷・製本　美研プリンティング株式会社

ISBN978-4-8079-0817-2
Printed in Japan

無断複写，転載を禁じます．本書添付の CD は，
図書館での非営利無料の貸出しに利用できます．

プライマリー薬学シリーズ 1
薬学英語入門 CD付

日本薬学会 編

編集担当：入江徹美・金子利雄・河野 円・Eric M. Skier
竹内典子・中村明弘・堀内正子

B5判　144ページ　定価2940円

日本薬学会の薬学教育カリキュラムを検討する協議会が定めた"薬学準備教育ガイドライン"に準拠した薬学生のための英語の教科書．ヒヤリングのためのCD付．

薬学生・薬剤師のための
英会話ハンドブック

原　博・Eric M. Skier・渡辺朋子 著　CD付

新書判　2色刷　224ページ　定価3150円

薬局や病院で薬剤師が，英語圏の患者に対応するときに役立つ実践的な英会話集．OTC薬の販売，受診勧告，服薬指導，病棟での治療薬の説明など実際の場面に沿った会話例を豊富に収載．ネイティブスピーカーにより主要スキットを録音した付録CDは，発音練習に役立つ．

看護師のための
英会話ハンドブック

上鶴重美・Eric M. Skier 著　CD付

新書判　2色刷　192ページ　定価1890円

病院で看護師が，英語圏の患者に対応するときに役立つ実践的な英会話集．外来・病棟・検査室・手術室といった多様な看護場面を取上げ，各場面でよく使う表現と英語のコツを学べるように，実際の場面に沿った会話例を豊富に掲載．聞き取りや発声練習に役立つネイティブスピーカーが録音した音声CDを進呈．

価格は税込 (2013年6月現在)